Biopolitics and the 'Obesity Epidemic'

Routledge Studies in Health and Social Welfare

Biopolitics and the 'Obesity Epidemic'

Governing Bodies

Edited by Jan Wright and Valerie Harwood

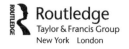

Routledge
Taylor & Francis Group
New York   London

First published 2009
by Routledge
711 Third Avenue, New York, NY 10017

Simultaneously published in the UK
by Routledge
2 Park Square, Milton Park, Abingdon, Oxon OX14 4RN

Routledge is an imprint of the Taylor & Francis Group, an informa business

First issued in paperback 2012

© 2009 Taylor & Francis

Typeset in Sabon by IBT Global.

Library of Congress Cataloging in Publication Data

Biopolitics and the "obesity epidemic" : governing bodies / edited by Jan Wright & Valerie Harwood.
   p. ; cm. — (Routledge studies in health and social welfare ; 3)
   Includes bibliographical references and index.
  1. Obesity—Social aspects. 2. Biopolitics. 3. Discourse analysis. I. Wright, Jan, 1948- II. Harwood, Valerie, 1967- III. Series.
[DNLM: 1. Obesity—epidemiology—Canada. 2. Obesity—epidemiology—United States. 3. Public Policy—Canada. 4. Public Policy—United States. 5. Research—Canada. 6. Research—United States. WD 210 B6156 2009]
  RA645.O23B56 2009
  362.196'398—dc22
  2008037539

ISBN13: 978–0-415–99188–9 (hbk)
ISBN13: 978–0-415–54094–0 (pbk)
ISBN13: 978–0-203–88206–1 (ebk)

Contents

PART II
Governing Young People:
Schools, Families and the 'Obesity Epidemic'

Part III: Commentary

Part I

Biopolitics and the 'Obesity Epidemic'

1 Biopower, Biopedagogies and the Obesity Epidemic

Jan Wright

One of the most powerful and pervasive discourses currently influencing ways of thinking about health and about bodies is that of the 'obesity epidemic'. This has, in turn, generated a counter argument from a range of perspectives. While there has been considerable recent theorising of the issue in the context of fat studies, there has been less attention to how the discourses associated with the obesity epidemic have had an impact on populations and specific sections of populations. The contributors to this book came together because of a joint concern as educators with the ways in which the 'truths' of the obesity epidemic, as they are recontextualized in government policy, health promotion initiatives, web resources and school practices have consequences for how children and young people come to know themselves. Our purpose then is to further current theoretical understandings of obesity discourse, and the practices it endorses, by interrogating what we are terming biopedagogical practices as they are enacted across a range of social and institutional sites. In bringing together collaborative insights around biopedagogies, the collection will also further theoretical understandings of the construction of the body in contemporary culture.

The starting point for this anthology is the argument that the 'obesity epidemic' and its associated practices depend on a range of pedagogies that affect contemporary life at both the level of the individual and the population. The notion of biopedagogies is drawn from Foucault's (1984) concept of 'biopower', the governance and regulation of individuals and populations through practices associated with the body. We use the term biopedagogies to describe the normalising and regulating practices in schools and disseminated more widely through the web and other forms of media, which have been generated by escalating concerns over claims of global 'obesity epidemic'. Through each of the chapters, this book makes the argument that biopedagogies not only place individuals under constant surveillance, but also press them towards increasingly monitoring themselves, often through increasing their *knowledge* around 'obesity' related risks, and 'instructing' them on how to eat healthily, and stay active. These systems of control can become constant within a 'totally pedagogized society' (Bernstein 2001) where methods to evaluate, monitor and survey the body are encouraged across a range of contemporary cultural practices including popular media (Burrows and Wright 2007) and new technologies (e.g., the Internet, see Miah and Rich 2008). In effect, individuals are being offered a number of ways to *understand* themselves, *change* themselves and *take action* to change others and their environments.

This first chapter serves as an introduction to the collection by describing the ideas that motivated the book. It begins by reviewing the literature that engages in a critical social analysis of the 'obesity epidemic' and its impact on individuals and populations, as a way of taking stock of the debate. It discusses the ways in which the debate and the theorising of the 'obesity epidemic' and related areas can move forward and how the resources of social theory can be marshalled to produce a counter discourse to that which dominates the media and current policy. The chapter explains the concept of biopedagogies and leads into chapter two, which expands on the notion of biopower and its utility in understanding the phenomenon of the 'obesity epidemic' and its effects.

THE PROBLEM OF THE 'OBESITY EPIDEMIC'

The idea that there is an 'obesity epidemic' has gained considerable purchase in the scientific health community and the public consciousness. This seems to have begun in the late 1990s with the publication of papers pointing to obesity as a serious health issue; one of these papers labelled the dramatic increase in people with a BMI above 30 between 1991 and 1998 as an 'epidemic' (Saguy and Almeling 2008). Mass media coverage has escalated from this point to where news articles (reporting on research alone) exceed 6,000 per year (Saguy and Almeling 2008). The issue of the 'obesity epidemic' has become a key plank in western (and increasingly Asian) governments' health agendas and worthy of front page reporting when new research is released. For example, in June 2008, a report that childhood obesity numbers were *not* increasing, from an Australian nutrition researcher, Jenny O'Dea (Creswell 2008), made it to the front page of the national newspaper, *The Australian*. While it is encouraging that counter arguments are being published, the article could only make sense as front-page news if the notion of 'childhood obesity' had already taken hold in the public consciousness as a matter of widespread interest. In comparison to this article, most media coverage, however, has been clearly instructive that there *is* an 'obesity epidemic', childhood obesity is particularly of concern, and that there is a clear relationship between weight and health, which affects individuals and the nation via economic costs. As Saguy and Almeling (2008) point out, the results of research reported in academic journals, which may be more tentative in suggesting these relationships, is taken up in government reports and newspapers in ways that single out and simplify to produce the most dramatic message. For example, Evans points to the certainty and hyperbole with which the House of Commons' (HOC) *Health Select Committee Report on Obesity* states that 'with quite astonishing rapidity, an epidemic of obesity has swept over England' and

> Should the gloomier scenarios relating to obesity turn out to be true, the sight of amputees will become much more familiar in the streets of Britain. There will be more blind people . . . [and] this will be the first generation where people die before their parents as a consequence of childhood obesity.
>
> (HOC 2006 quoted in Evans 2006: 262)

As many have pointed out, including writers in this book, the naming of obesity as a disease, and the identification of specific risk factors provides the impetus for the close monitoring of those who might be at risk in the name of prevention, and the assumed need for treatment of those who fall within the medically defined categories of overweight or obesity. This has been given further purchase by the moral opprobrium directed at those who are perceived (through the reading of their bodies) not to be making appropriate lifestyle decisions and thereby abandoning their responsibilities (and therefore their rights) as citizens contributing to the general good. As is developed further in the following chapters, the taken for granted relationship between weight and health, and its apparent costs to individuals and society, also provides the motivation and mechanisms for the recontextualization of bio-medical knowledge in reports that can be used to both argue for the need for public education and provide the content for that education. For example, in January 2008 the British government outlined a new strategy, including a £75 million, 3-year advertising campaign that called for an 'evidence-based marketing program which will inform, support and empower parents in making changes to their children's diet and levels of physical activity' (Department of Health 2008). Other examples of public health education campaigns include *Mission On* (New Zealand), *2 and 5* (Australia), ParticipACTION (Canada) and a national campaign in Japan for mandatory measurement of the waist circumferences of all people aged between 40 and 75 (Onishi 2008). These campaigns provide the public with the facts about the obesity epidemic, the likely health and economic effects, and instructions on how to act to protect themselves and their children from such effects.

There has been for many years, a critique of western societies' 'cult of slenderness' and an examination of its effects for how people, and women in particular regard themselves and their bodies. Alongside and informed by this writing there has also been a fat activist movement that has gained momentum with the advent of the Internet (see Saguy and Riley 2005). However, it has only been with the public and bio-medical focus on obesity and the relationship between weight and health that the discourse has taken a different turn to provoke a proliferation of responses, from a range of different perspectives; some of which have found the apparent compatibility of their arguments distinctly unsettling (see Chapter 3, this volume).

The phenomenon of what Saguy and Riley (2005) have called anti-obesity research and activism has marshalled a counter 'movement', from a range of perspectives including the bio-sciences, social sciences, and cultural studies. Those on the 'other' side of the debate have been categorized by Saguy and Riley as fat activist researchers (such as Paul Campos and Paul Ernsberger) and fat acceptance activists (such as the National Association to Advance Fat Acceptance (NAAFA). I maintain, however, that this categorisation (which worked very well for the purpose of their analysis of the debate) elides the important differences in purposes and positions that motivate what is a more complex collection of, mostly but not always, likeminded people (see Chapter 3 as an example). I would argue that while most want to challenge the 'truths' of the obesity epidemic, not all would align seamlessly with fat activism, which is in itself not a singular position (see Lebesco 2004), nor vice versa.

Social and cultural researchers, however, often rely heavily (see the introductions to many of the chapters in this book) on those who have taken on the bio-scientists and epidemiologists in their own territory, because it seems this is a terrain on which there can be a common language. The critique of the science that supports the attention given to the obesity epidemic and its relationship with health has been gaining momentum in the public and academic domain (but as yet with little apparent purchase at the level of government) since the publication of a number of books and several articles in academic, medical and health journals (Campos 2004; Campos, Saguy, Ernsberger, Oliver and Gaesser 2006; Flegal 2005; Gard and Wright 2005). These scholars and scientists examine the 'science' of the 'obesity epidemic' on its own terms, challenging the propositions on scientific criteria of 'truth'—for example, quality of the methodology, the interpretations and theorising from the data—and pointing to studies that provide alternative understandings. As these scholars point out, the research that would support the claim of an 'obesity epidemic' and the importance of overweight and obesity to health is far from conclusive (e.g., Campos et al. 2006; Gard and Wright 2005; Mark 2005) and certainly much less certain than we are led to believe in the media and by government policies and initiatives. Some of the criticisms include: the easy conflation between obesity and overweight in the use of the term 'obesity'; the use of the very blunt instrument of the Body Mass Index (BMI) as a measure of overweight and obesity; and the claims made about the causal relationship between overweight and obesity and a wide range of diseases (see Gard and Wright 2005 and Jutel and Halse in this book). Criticisms are also levelled at the claims made about the relationship between children's behaviour (watching television, playing computers, generally lying around, the 'couch potato' rhetoric that regularly occurs in media and also in children's language) and their weight (see Biddle, Gorely, Marshall, Murdey and Cameron 2004; Gard and Wright 2005; Marshall, Biddle, Sallis, McKenzie and Conway 2002).

Despite a proliferation of papers and books in the social sciences and cultural studies (and indeed, as demonstrated above, from within the 'bio-physical sciences') critiquing the idea of an 'obesity epidemic' and its effects, nowhere is the divide between the bio-physical and medical sciences and socioculturally informed research and theorising more evident than around this issue. Nor is the power of science to establish the normative position more clearly demonstrated. Whereas those who would interrogate the knowledge constructed in the name of obesity science have to take considerable care with their claims and constantly defend their positions, those speaking from the standpoint of science have no such qualms, rarely engaging with the debates, dismissing the research by questioning the credibiltiy of authors (as non-scientists or non-medical researchers) and/ or using derogatory epithets to dismiss alternative positions. As Saguy and Riley (2005: 870) argue, on the basis of their analysis of the claims from both sides of the debate, the central role played by morality in the debate, together with medical arguments about the risks of body weight, 'stymie rights claims and justify morality-based fears'.

The critiques of the 'truths' of the obesity epidemic are important, especially in domains where social and cultural arguments have less purchase. In this book, however, we draw on social theory to address different questions. We look to Foucault, in particular, but also other social theorists, such as Bernstein, Bulter and Deleuze and those who have used their work in the area of critical health sociology, to make visible the ways the ideas or discourse associated with the obesity epidemic work to govern bodies and to provide the social meanings by which individuals come to know themselves and others. The point of this book is not to argue with the scientific 'truths' (there are others who have taken up this task). Rather it is to demonstrate how these 'truths' become 'recontextualized' in different social and cultural sites to inform and persuade people on how they should understand their bodies and how they should live their lives. In doing so, in this chapter, I look to those who have drawn our attention to the importance of such a pursuit, who have pointed to the body as more than its biology, but as a site where social meanings become embodied and in doing so change 'consciousness', identities or subjectivities (depending on your theoretical bent). What Christine Halse, in this collection, following Deleuze, describes as 'the incorporation of the "outside" world (the social and economic well-being of others) into "inside" (psyche and body) of the individual'.

ACKNOWLEDGING THE FEMINIST CONTRIBUTION

Although the term 'obesity' has now captured public attention, the implications of a social and cultural preoccupation with body size and shape and appearance have been the focus of social theorists (for example, Mike Featherstone) and particularly feminists for some decades (for example, Andrea

Dworkin, Susan Bartky, Naomi Woolf, Susan Orbach, Kim Chernin to name a few). Prompted by a concern with the increasing evidence of eating disorders amongst young women, feminists made the link between social structures, cultural ideals and the body, particularly, in this case, the female body.

This early work of feminism seems frequently to be elided in oft cited concerns of the loss of the fleshyness of the body in contemporary critiques of poststructuralist theorising of the body (Shilling 2008). Feminists such as Dworkin (cited in Bordo 2003) and later Bordo, however, were very much concerned with the relationship between material bodies and 'the "direct grip" culture has on our bodies through the practices and bodily habits of everyday life' (2003: 16). Bordo acknowledges her debt to early feminists, such as Mary Wollestencraft, who through their own experiences and politicization theorized the ways culture is not simply written on to but shapes both the body, body comportment and through this process women's conciousness. These ideas resonate with contempory writing around fat bodies; the themes of alienation and self-loathing and the the processes by which particular kinds of body real or imaginary become constituted as abject (Kristeva 1982 and see Murray in this book).

Bordo (2003: 32) draws on Foucault to point to the micropractices, what we might call biopedagogies, that are a 'constant and intimate fact of everyday life': the self-assessment, self-monitoring of bodies and behaviours against social norms of appearance and body shape and the moral imperatives regarding eating and exercise (so called 'lifestyle' behaviours). She argues that there is a '[desperate need for] the critical edge of a systemic perspective' which focuses on the 'institutionalized system of values and practices within which girls and women—and, increasingly, boys and men as well—come to believe they are nothing (and frequently treated as nothing) unless they are trim, tight, lineless, bulgeless, and sagless' (p.32).

The focus in the early feminist writing on the body was primarily on anorexia and eating disorders and the ways the preoccupation with the body, evidenced in the numbers of young women diagnosed with eating discorders, was part of the experience and self-consiousness of most girls and women in western societies. That analysis continues, inflected now with an analysis of culture in which health is equated with weight and where moral imperatives associated with the moral panic of the 'obesity epidemic' add another dimension to an already complex issue. As Halse and Rich and Evans in this book suggest desires to be thin need also to be understood in a neoliberal and performative culture where individuals are expected to be responsible not only for their own health but for striving for perfection in all aspects of their lives, including the weight and appearance of their bodies. To be fat (however that is perceived by society and/or the individual) is evidence of failure.

Queering Fat/Fat Activism

The naming of fat 'as a feminist issue' has promoted another line of social analysis and activism. This is primarily informed by feminist theory and increasingly by cultural studies and particularly queer theory, for example, see Braziel and Lebesco (2001), Lebesco (2001, 2004) and also Murray (2005 and in this collection). Promotion of a notion of 'body diversity' underpins the arguments of most proponents of this position, but as Lebesco (2004) argues in her final chapter of *Revolting Bodies*, some proponents are more willing to take up health arguments than others. Some fat activists will use the notion of obesity as a disease determined by genes in order to argue that, being biological, it is not their fault that they are fat and therefore they should not be the target of moral judgements nor discrimination. Much of the early writing and continuing research in this field analyses western society's relationship with fat and fat bodies and seeks to make visible the experience of women who judge themselves and are judged as overweight (e.g., Carryer 1997; Davies 1998). These researchers point to the damaging effects on fat women of social stigmatisation and discrimination. They often seek to address commonly held prejudices that people are fat because they are not strong willed enough, because they haven't tried hard enough, that is, it is all their own fault.

More recently queer theory (and particulary Judith Butler) has been used to provoke, and to name the discourses that constitute fat and fat bodies as abject. For example in their introduction to *Bodies out of Bounds*, Brazeil and Lebesco (2001: 1) write: '[o]ne of the objectives, then, is unmasking the fat body, rendering it visible and present, rather than invisible and absent: seen rather than unsightly'. Lebesco (2004: 3) goes further in *Revolting Bodies* to move aesthetic and health constructions of fat into a political domain; her interest is in 'transforming fatness from a spoiled, uninhabitable, invisible identity to a stronger subject position'. Her project is to resignify the fat body 'as healthy and powerful' and to provide the resources (the ways of thinking) to resist stigmatising messages from anti-fat. In the terms of this book, she and others (see Murray in this collection) are attempting to disrupt the comfortable social understandings of fat and obesity and provide others ways of knowing to inform the way people live their bodies and how they regard and relate to their own and the bodies of others.

BIOPEDAGOGY(IES)

We use the word biopedagogies in this book to bring together the idea of biopower and pedagogy in ways that help us understand the the body as a political space. This accentuates the meanings associated with the body and how these are constituted in multiple 'pedagogical sites'—that is, sites that have the power to teach, to engage 'learners' in meaning making practices that they use to make sense of their worlds and their selves and thereby influence how they act on themselves and others. These sites are not necessarily (and indeed mostly) in schools, but are everywhere around us, on the web, on television, radio and film, billboards and posters, and pamphlets in doctors' waiting rooms. Some are deliberate attempts to change behaviour, such as the public health campaigns associated with the 'obesity epidemic', others are more subtle and perhaps because of this more powerful. For example, reality TV shows such as *The Greatest Loser* and *Honey We're Killing the Kids* promote the idea that change is absolutely necessary and that to not change is unthinkable—'your children will die'—and inexcusable—the competitors on *The Greatest Loser* demonstrate for all to see that it is possible to lose large amounts of weight. These shows are the most direct in their message, but similar messages about risk, lifestyles and individual responsibility are evident in the presentation of health issues in radio commentary, daily popular soaps and the ways in which fatness and large people are characterized in film and television. These spaces also provide opportunities for rebellion and resistance, both explicity by different representatins of fat women and men (see Lebesco's analysis of these in *Revolting Bodies*), but also through the public discussions they provoke about ways of seeing fatness.

Bordo uses the word pedagogy in the introduction to the 2003 edition of *Unbearable Weight* to write about the power of digitally altered media images in teaching us how to see the 'ideal body',

> This [digitally modified images of "virtually every celebrity image"] is not just a matter of deception—boring old stuff, which ads have traded on from their beginnings. This is perceptual pedagogy, How to Interpret Your Body 101. These images are teaching us how to see.
>
> (Bordo 2003: xviii)

As a term 'pedagogy' has been taken to mean many different things. Following Lusted's (1986) influential paper in *Screen* it has had the potential to go beyond a simple notion of transmission, to understand pedagogy as a relational cultural practice through which knowledge is produced. It is a practice that involves the negotiation of knowledge (ideas) in relations of power and one that goes beyond the classroom. Most recently following Basil Bernstein, Evans, Rich, Davies and Allwood (2008: 17) have argued that pedagogy encompasses all those ubiquitous (conscious) practices which would instruct about how one should live; these are always value laden and 'help lay down the rules of belonging to a culture and class'. Body pedagogies, from their point of view, then are 'any conscious activity [under]taken by people, organisations or the state, that are designed to enhance individuals' understandings of their own and others' corporeality'.

In going beyond the notion of body pedagogies—as pedagogies that target the body—we draw on Foucault's concept of biopower (see Harwood in Chapter 2 for a detailed discussion) to conceive of the body as inextricably bound up with life (or bios). This enables us to understand biopedagogies as those disciplinary and regulatory strategies that enable the governing of bodies in the name of health and life. The cojoining of biopower and pedagogy allows us to suggest a framework for the analysis of 'biopedagogical practices. These practices produce the truths associated with the obesity epidemic and include for example, the 'strategies for intervention', the power relations and modes of instruction across a wide range of social and instituitional sites, enacted in the name of the 'obesity epidemic'. Biopedagogies can be understood as urging people to work on themselves. However, as the authors in this book point out, this is not always predictable. How individuals take up ideas around fatness and obesity will be mediated by their personal experiences, their own embodiment, their interactions with other ways of knowing, other truths and operations of power in relation to the knowledge produced around health, obesity and the body.

THE CHAPTERS

The book is divided into two sections with a commentary by Valerie Walkerdine completing the collection. Part I takes a more theoretical stance examining how particular obesity discourses have come into being and how these are circulating—normalising, regulating and so on—to govern populations. Part II of the book focuses on how ideas associated with the obesity epidemic contribute to the governing of the population through specific biopedagogies or interventions. Most of the chapters draw on empirical work to examine the truths of the obesity epidemic, particularly the ways in which they have been recontextualized in school and public health interventions that target families and young people. Part I begins with a key chapter in which Valerie Harwood explains how drawing on Foucault's notions of biopower and an understanding of pedagogy as a relation between knowledge and individuals in the context of particular social sites enables us to exceed the theoretical potential of each, particularly in the analysis of the ways in which ideas about obesity are taken up, transmitted and resisted by individuals, institutions, and governments.

In Chapter 3 Michael Gard makes an important and provocative contribution by challenging critical obesity researchers and fat activists, including the contributors to this book, to beware of complacency with their/our own positions. He argues that, if we to have more public effect, we need to be open to understanding how other intellectual traditions operate and to use these strategically to speak in languages other than those with which we are comfortable; that is, we should not let the well worn grooves of our own discursive positions inhibit our capacity to speak to many different audiences. He also suggests that we need to more closely interrogate the invested positions of those whose ideas we would take up because they seem to support our arguments and those who would use our arguments to support positions that may be counter to our own.

The remaining writers in this section examine how the medicalization of weight through its association with health, becomes a key component of public health discourses of individual responsibility, morality and the drawing up of distinctions between the normal and the pathological. They each examine the processes by which these truths come into being and the power they derive from an association between health and morality. They bring to the surface those ideas about obesity and fat that are hard to contest, to speak against. These chapters make visible this process, both through exemplification/illustration and by drawing on robust theory to say why this is a problem. They point to how the uncontested re-citation of ways of talking and acting on bodies in the name of the obesity epidemic are dangerous and offer other ways of knowing and acting.

In Chapter 5, Annemarie Jutel explores the genesis of the medical position on overweight and obesity through an analysis of the 'convergence of conditions which have led to the consideration of overweight as a disease'. These include the ways the appearance of the body has come to signify the worth of the individual; and the capacity to measure fatness, to establish an objective truth about a person's weight. The idea that the social and personal worth of a person is indicated by their appearance is taken further by Samantha Murray and Christine Halse in their chapters in Part I. They both develop the idea that the obesity discourse is charged with notions of morality and virtue, where appearance is indicative of not only an individual's lifestyle practices, their attitudes and choices but also of their relationship to the good of the rest of their society and their cost to that society. Murray draws attention to John Burry's argument that maintaining a 'healthy' weight is not only the responsibility of individuals but is also a matter of ethics. Halse develops this idea in her description of the moral imperatives associated with weight control as a 'virtue discourse'. She argues that what sets virtue discourses apart from other discourses is the way they 'configure virtue as an open-ended condition: a state of excellence that has no boundaries or exclusions' (Halse, Honey and Boughtwood 2007: 220).

In Part II of the book, the authors describe how the truths of the obesity epidemic are recontextualized as 'strategies for intervention . . . in the name of life and health' (Rabinow and Rose 2006: 196). Remarkably similar interventions encouraging populations to make 'responsible' decisions in relation to eating and physical activity have proliferated across the United States, Canada, the United Kingdom, Australia and New Zealand (and more recently in Japan, Hong Kong and Singapore). These normalize particular practices with the apparent imprimatur of science and demonize others and by doing so normalize particular ways of living and being. In the process, they contribute to other individualising discourses that would blame particular social groups for their failure to live up to social standards of health. These interventions and the moral ideas of individual responsibility for one's health that underpin them provide a context in which measuring weight, calculating the BMI, comparing these measures against standards and the monitoring of eating and activity as part of everyday and institutionalized practice become acceptable. The discourses of the obesity epidemic are enacted on the bodies of children and young people in schools, in patient consultations in doctors' surgeries and by individuals on themselves via the mechanisms for self-monitoring offered on the web, in popular magazines and similar popular media sites.

Importantly, the authors in Part II demonstrate how these interventions are targeted specifically at families, young people and children. While Murray and Halse draw our attention to how bodies become abject in the context of the obesity discourses, in Part II, in the chapters by Lisette Burrows and Laura Azzarito, we see how the obesity discourses are used in conjunction with racialized and classed discourses to mobilize feelings of blame and disgust around whole populations (e.g. poor, working class, cultural minorities). Burrows demonstrates how Maori and Pacifika peoples in New Zealand through media coverage of obesity are constituted as being at greater risk of obesity, and of the health consequences assumed to be associated with it, through what are described as their 'inappropriate' cultural practices and values around eating and exercise.

Azzarito in her chapter argues that the normative discourses of the obesity epidemic privilege white gendered ideas of the fit healthy body and white cultural practices associated with eating and activity and thereby constitute the cultural practices and the non-white bodies of marginalized people of colour as 'Other'. She examines specific school-based research interventions in the United States aimed at improving the health of young African American, Hispanic and Native American people and argues that these are narrowly based on racialized categories of healthy and fit bodies, that they contribute to the 'reclaiming of race as a biological category' and to the assimilation of 'the bodies of young people from different ethnic background to whiteness'.

As Deana Leahy points out in her chapter, governmental regulation is not only about drawing on expert knowledge to set up particular ways of living but also about the way affect is mobilized in the process of subjectification. As she says so evocatively, the pedagogies invoked in health classrooms in the name of teaching about bodies, nutrition and health, 'are explicitly designed to permeate and creep into students' ways of thinking and being'. She describes, through data collected in classrooms, how students are invited via biopedagogical strategies to understand themselves and their bodies in relation to particular expert understandings of fitness and health. More importantly, however, are the ways in which expert knowledge is mobilized by the teacher in her talk about the relationship between exercise, fitness and fat, to elicit bodily responses, and in particular in Leahy's examples, disgust. Leahy argues that 'disgust' is an affect commonly mobilized by both teachers and students in health classes and by other health strategies designed to address childhood obesity.

In their chapters, Natalie Beausoleil, Simone Fullagar, Geneviève Rail, Emma Rich and John Evans use interviews with families or young people to demonstrate how the health imperatives associated with the obesity epidemic, as promoted through government and school interventions are taken up by families and young people in the way they talk about their bodies, their health and their lives. Fullagar, for example, examines the texts of health promotion initiatives directed at preventing obesity alongside the texts from interviews with families about their decision-making practices around health. She demonstrates the power of the health promotion discourses in the ways the families talked about health, in how they negotiated risks and how feelings of shame and despair influenced their decision-making. Her analysis exemplifies the way the 'lived body' is the site of a discursive struggle where competing meanings of health and lifestyle decisions are made in relation to material circumstances and the relational contexts of families.

Rich and Evans use the *Every Child Matters* policy document to identify techniques of surveillance, which in the name of informing young people (and their parents, through measuring their child's weight online) about their health produce affects such as anxiety, stress and guilt. They argue that these reach into every aspect of young people's lives both inside and outside schools, through the moral imperatives to be a particular kind of person. These also provide teachers and health educators (and, I would argue, friends, family and sometimes only nodding acquaintances) with the assumed right to make moral judgements on young people's bodies and to become expert in recommending how they should eat, exercise and generally live their lives in order to lose or maintain a 'healthy weight'. They draw on their interviews with young women diagnosed with anorexia to demonstrate the damaging effects of such regulatory techniques. For example many of the young people they interviewed talked about such techniques (such as being weighed in class) as critical moments in how they came to view their bodies.

Geneviève Rail and Natalie Beausoleil also draw on interviews with young people, this time from a large study investigating the meanings of health and fitness for Canadian young people. Both Rail and Beausoleil demonstrate the power of the obesity discourse in promoting particular 'truths' about exercise, eating, energy balance and appearance to persuade young people to particular ways of knowing their bodies, no matter what their ethnic or social class background. Beausoleil, writing from the position of a feminist and health activist in the area of body image and prevention of eating disorders, documents the difficulties for activists in the face of public health messages and school initiatives premised on the moral assumptions of very powerful regulatory discourses of 'health' and the 'healthy body'. Like other writers in this collection she also points to spaces for resistance and opportunities for social change, in her case, through concerns around increasing incidences of young people diagnosed with eating disorders and the desire by officials to 'do no harm'.

All of the authors in this collection use resources of social theory and their empirical work to reveal how, via biopedagogies, the truths associated with 'obesity epidemic' are produced. This provides the key to thinking through ways of countering a discourse that equates health with weight and produces ways of thinking about and acting on bodies that are detrimental to the well-being of individuals and populations. From a poststructuralist position there is no escaping discourse, nor the processes of truth making and the defining of subjects that this implies. However, taking up Foucault, we can contest the truths and the relations of power in which they are produced (Harwood 2006). The truths associated with the 'obesity epidemic' and the interventions promoted in the name of addressing the obesity problem, as argued by the authors in this collection, do not contribute to the health of populations; rather they divide populations on the basis of moral judgements about appearance, weight and lifestyle decisions, with effects that are damaging to individuals and groups. Moreover, whole populations are interpellated (Althusser 1971) by the discourse so that individuals, families, institutions make decisions about their lives and those for whom they are responsible on basis of the 'risk' of obesity that might occur. The effectiveness of the discourse is its capacity to engage the emotions of shame, guilt and fear, not only amongst those who are already defined as 'abject' (following Kristeva 1982) or 'not normal' but for all in the fear that they might become so. By pointing out how the discourse works we hope by this book to provide alternative 'truths', resources for different ways of knowing, and different ways of understanding health, selves and bodies.

REFERENCES

Althusser, L. (1971) *Lenin and Philosophy*, New York: Monthly Review Press.
Bernstein, B. (2001) 'From Pedagogies to Knowledges', in A. Morais, I. Neves, B. Davies and H. Daniels (eds) *Towards a Sociology of Pedagogy. The Contribution of Basil Bernstein to Research*, New York: Peter Lang.
Biddle, S.J.H., Gorely, T., Marshall, S.J., Murdey, I. and Cameron, N. (2004) 'Physical activity and sedentary behaviours in youth: issues and controversies', *Journal of the Royal Society for the Promotion of Health*, 124(1): 29–33.
Bordo, S. (2003) *Unbearable Weight: Feminism, Western Culture and the Body*, 10th edn, Berkeley: University of California Press.
Braziel, J.E. and Lebesco, K. (eds) (2001) *Bodies Out of Bounds: Fatness and Transgression*, Berkeley: University of California Press.
Burrows, L. and Wright, J. (2007) 'Prescribing practices: shaping healthy children in schools', *International Journal of Children's Rights*, 15: 83–98.
Campos, P. (2004) *The Obesity Myth: Why America's Obsession with Weight is Hazardous to your Health*, New York: Penguin Books.
Campos, P., Saguy, A., Ernsberger, P., Oliver, E. and Gaesser, G. (2006) 'The epidemiology of overweight and obesity: public health crisis or moral panic?', *International Journal of Epidemiology*, 35(1): 55–60.
Carryer, J. (1997) 'The embodied experience of largeness: a feminist exploration', in V. Grace and M. de Ras (eds) *Bodily Boundaries, Sexualised Genders and Medical Discourses*, Palmerston North: Dunmore Press.
Cresswell, A. (2008) 'Hysteria over fat children inflated', *The Weekend Australian*, May 31: retrieved 16 June 2008, from http://www.theaustralian.news.com.au/story/0,25197,23786484-601,00.html

Davies, D. (1998) 'Health and the Discourse of Weight Control', in A. Petersen and C. Waddell (eds) *Health Matters: A Ssociology of Illness, Prevention and Care*, Buckingham, UK: Open University Press.

Department of Health (2008) *Healthy Weight, Healthy Lives: A Cross- Government Strategy for England*, retrieved 18 June 2008, from http://www.dh.gov.uk/en/Publichealth/Healthimprovement/Obesity/DH_082383

Evans, B. (2006) '"Gluttony or sloth": critical geographies of bodies in (anti)obesity policy', *Area*, 38(3), 259–67.

Evans, J., Rich, E., Davies, B. and Allwood, R. (2008) *Education, Eating Disorders and Obesity Discourse: Fat Fabrication*, London and New York: Routledge.

Flegal, K.M., Graubard, B.I., Williamson, D.F. and Gail, M.H. (2005) 'Excess deaths associated with underweight, overweight, and obesity', *Journal of the American Medical Association*, 293(15): 1861–7.

Foucault, M. (1984) *The History of Sexuality, Volume I: An Introduction*, Harmondsworth, Middlesex, England: Peregrine, Penguin Books.

Gard, M. and Wright, J. (2005) *The 'Obesity Epidemic': Science, Ideology and Morality*, London: Routledge.

Halse, C., Honey, A., and Boughtwood, D. (2007) 'The paradox of virtue: (re) thinking deviance, anorexia and schooling', *Gender and Education*, 19(2): 219–35.

Harwood, V. (2006) *Diagnosing Disorderly Children*, London: Routledge.

Kristeva, J. (1982) *Powers of Horror: An Essay in Abjection*, New York: Columbia University Press.

Lebesco, K. (2001) 'Queering Fat Bodies/Politics', in J.E. Braziel and K. Lebesco (eds) *Bodies Out of Bounds: Fatness and Transgression*, Berkeley: University of California Press.

Lebesco, K. (2004) *Revolting Bodies: The Struggle to Redefine Fat Identity*, Amherst and Boston: University of Massachusetts Press.

Lusted, D. (1986) 'Why pedagogy', *Screen*, 27(5): 2–15.

Mark, D. (2005) 'Deaths attributable to obesity', *Journal of the American Medical Association*, 293(15): 1918–19.

Marshall, S.J., Biddle, S.J.H., Sallis, J.F., McKenzie, I.L. and Conway, T.L. (2002) 'Clustering of sedentary behaviours and physical activity among youth: a cross-national study', *Paediatric Exercise Science*, 14: 401–7.

Miah, A. and Rich, E. (2008) *The Medicalisation of Cyberspace*, New York: Routledge.

Murray, S. (2005) '(Un/be)coming out? Rethinking fat politics', *Social Semiotics*, 15(2), 153–163.

Onishi, N. (2008) 'Japan, seeking trim waists, measures millions', *New York Times*, Asia Pacific, June 13: retrieved 18 June 2008, from http://www.nytimes.com/2008/06/13/world/asia/13fat.html?_r=2andno_interstitialandoref=slogin

Rabinow, P. and Rose, N. (2006) 'Biopower today', *BioSocieties*, 1: 195–217.

Saguy, A.C. and Riley, K. (2005) 'Weighing both sides: morality, mortality, and framing contests over obesity', *Journal of Health Politics, Policy and Law*, 30(5): 869–921.

Saguy, A. and Almeling, R. (2008) 'Fat in the fire? Science, the news media, and the "obesity epidemic?"', *Sociological Forum*, 23(1): 53–83.

Shilling, C. (2008) 'Foreword: Body Pedagogics, Society and Schooling', in J. Evans, E. Rich, B. Davies and R. Allwood (eds) *Education, Disordered Eating and Obesity Discourse: Fat Fabrications*, London: Routledge.

2 Theorizing Biopedagogies

Valerie Harwood

INTRODUCTION

Across a range of contemporary contexts are instructions on *bios*: how to live, how to eat, how much to eat, how to move, how much to move. In short an extensive pedagogy is aimed at us: a pedagogy of *bios*, or what can be termed 'biopedagogy'. This biopedagogy is premised on a conflation between *bios* and health where there is far more at stake than simply 'being well'. As the chapters in this collection point out, the effectiveness of the 'obesity epidemic' in influencing beliefs, behaviours, and health and educational policies is very much tied to these practices that we are terming biopedagogy.

'Biopedagogies' draws inspiration from Michel Foucault's articulation of biopower. The concept of 'biopower' has been taken up by several researchers in the area of health, including Denise Gastaldo (1997) who has argued for a conceptualization of health education as biopower. Biopower has been drawn on in health related areas, such as psychotherapy (Hook 2003), therapy and renal failure (Holmes, Perron, and Savoi 2006) and facilitated reproduction via egg donors (Pollock 2003), and Nikolas Rose (2006) has examined biopower and pharmogenomics. There remains however, the question as to how to explicate a conceptual approach to the analysis of biopower, and in turn, how to translate this into methodological practices that can interrogate the empirical. A recent paper by Paul Rabinow and Nikolas Rose (2006: 197) intervenes in this space by offering an outline of biopower's 'plane of actuality.'[1] In this chapter I draw closely on this work to develop the concept of biopedagogies, and suggest some ways forward for interrogating the pedagogical practices and effects of biopower, and how in our contemporary contexts these practices work to govern bodies.

BIOPOWER

Foucault's discussion of biopower occurs in the mid-1970s in the *History of Sexuality Volume One* (1984) published in French in 1976 and in the 1975–76 Lectures *Society Must Be Defended* at the Collège de France

(2003). In these discussions Foucault draws attention to the change from sovereign power, one marked by a variation in the attention to life and death. As he writes in the opening lines of the last chapter of the *History of Sexuality*, 'one of the characteristic privileges of sovereign power was the right to decide life and death' (Foucault 1984: 135). In the final lecture of the 1975–76 course, Foucault points to the 'practical disequilibrium' of this power,

> The right of life and death is always exercised in an unbalanced way: the balance is always tipped in favor of death. Sovereign power's effect on life is exercised only when the sovereign can kill. The very essence of the right of life and death is actually the right to kill: it is at the moment when the sovereign can kill that he exercises his right over life.
>
> (Foucault 2003: 240)

Sovereign power is thus premised on the right to take life, it has power over life only insofar as it can 'let live'. This type of power 'was essentially a right of seizure: of things, time, bodies, and ultimately life itself; it culminated in the privilege to seize hold of life in order to suppress it' (Foucault 1984: 136).

Biopower has a starkly divergent concern: an emphasis on 'life'. When Foucault (2000) moves to discuss biopower, it is precisely this distinction that he draws on to characterize the changes of state control in the eighteenth and nineteenth centuries. Rather than a basis of 'taking life', the objective of biopower was to preserve life. Characterizing it as the 'opposite right' to sovereign power, this 'is the power to "make" live and "let" die' (Foucault 2003: 241). In this sense, rather than death as the moment where sovereign power enacts power, in biopower it is *life, or the power to conserve or protect life where power is enacted*. As Foucault (1984: 138) sums up, '[n]ow it is over life, throughout its unfolding, that power establishes its dominion; death is power's limit'.

This focus on life needs to be understood not as the heralding of some new caring and kinder age; but in terms of the aims of the state to solidify itself via the control of life (and hence strength, economic viability) of its population. Whilst Foucault (1984: 136) states that '[t]his death that was based on the right of the sovereign is now manifested as simply the reverse right of the social body to ensure, maintain, or develop its life', he quickly points out the extent of the wars, bloodshed, and genocide that have occurred alongside this rubric of 'life'. Indeed, in both sources (*The History of Sexuality Volume One* and the 1975–76 Lectures) Foucault makes the case that the claim of preserving life gave justification to racism, to killing members of a state's own population in the name of conserving the very life of that population.[2] This is the rub of biopower. It is a power that appears life conserving, yet functions to *fortify populations* in the name of modern state power, commanding practices in the name of life (and whether these are indeed life enhancing is open to debate). As such, the rising concerns with obesity need to be understood as linked with biopower, and the practices promulgating health measures can be conceived as biopedagogies of this biopower. But this is not to assume biopower, or rather technologies of biopower, are bad. Neither is it to characterize biopower as totalizing, to which there is no resistance, a point I take up later. Rather, as the chapters in this volume demonstrate, it is an invitation to look more carefully at how notions of obesity function as part of biopower. Read in this manner, penetrating questions can be posed of these practices and the ways in which we are 'taught', via biopedagogies, to be 'healthy' (and good) citizens.

Foucault (1984: 139) provides an outline of biopower that situates it as having two poles, the first of these is the *'anatomo-politics of the human body'*, while the 'second, [is] focused on the species body.'[3] Or to again quote Foucault (1984: 139), '[t]he disciplines of the body and the regulations of the population constituted the two poles around which the organization of power over life was deployed'. Describing the first pole as emerging in the seventeenth century, Foucault sees this as

> [T]echniques of power that were essentially centered on the body, on the individual body. They included all devices that were used to ensure the spatial distribution of individual bodies (their separation, their alignment, their serialization, and their surveillance) and the organization, around those individuals, of a whole field of visibility.
>
> (Foucault 2003: 242)

The techniques of power 'centered on the body, the *individual body*' (Foucault 2003: 242, emphasis added) were disciplinary.

> They were techniques for rationalizing and strictly economizing on a power that had to be used in the least costly way possible, thanks to a whole system of surveillance, hierarchies, inspections, bookkeeping, and reports—all the technology that can be described as the disciplinary technology of labor.
>
> (Foucault 2003: 242)

Discipline and Punish (Foucault 1991) provides an analysis of this form of power. The frequently cited technique of panopticism is an exemplar of such disciplinary technology; an economizing power centered on individual bodies seeking to render them docile.

In the 1975–76 Lectures Foucault (2003: 242) describes the second pole as 'emerging in the second half of the eighteenth century'. This pole varies from the first where '[u]nlike discipline, which is addressed to bodies, the new nondisciplinary power is applied not to man-as-body but to the living man, to man-as-living-being; ultimately if you like, to man-as-species' (Foucault 2003: 242). The focus here is on 'the multiplicity of men',

So after the first seizure of power over the body in an individualizing mode, we have a second seizure of power that is not individualizing but, if you like, massifying, that is directed not at man-as-body but at man-as-species.

(Foucault 2003: 243)

This breathes a rather different take on bios, where the individual-as-life becomes thoroughly allied with the population-as-life. Populations are invigilated via a 'technology of biopower . . . over "the" population as such, over men insofar as they are living beings. It is continuous, scientific, and it is the power to make live' (Foucault 2003: 247). Here power functions through regulation, it is regulatory, what Foucault calls 'the power of regularization'.

While the panopticon is emblematic of disciplinary power and its individualizing practices, it is the control of populations, the species via regulation by, for example public health that is illustrative of this second mode. This mode emphasizes 'the administration of bodies and the calculated management of life' (Foucault 1984: 139–40). Responding to this, we need to ask what are the positions at which this power over life operates? An indication lies in Foucault's (2003: 242) explanation that this 'technique exists at a different level, on a different scale, and because it has a different bearing area, and makes use of very different instruments'. These are instruments that can be put into effect to regularize the populations, a principal one of which is pedagogy.

These two poles, disciplinary power that focuses on individualization and regularizing power that focuses on massifying, work in a related fashion. Whilst the second pole is described as emerging later than the first, it is not the case that one replaced the other, or were 'antithetical . . . they constituted rather two poles of development linked together by a whole intermediary cluster of relations' (Foucault 1984: 139). What this second pole does is 'dovetail into it [the first pole], integrate it, modify it to some extent, and above all, use it by sort of infiltrating it, embedding itself in existing disciplinary techniques' (Foucault 2003: 242). Hook (2003: 616) adds to this perspective when he suggests that 'this conglomerate notion of "disciplinary bio-power" thus usefully enables Foucault to join "bottom-up" and "top-down" "flows" of power, whilst maintaining an emphasis on technical and tactical imperatives'.

Disciplinary power and regularizing power differ markedly from sovereign power. Firstly, whilst sovereign power may be thought of as 'repressive', these forms of power are *productive*. Productive power helps to explain the abundance of technologies and discourses that circulate, multiply, modify. This is apparent in the very things which 'mark[ed] the era of biopower', that is, the 'explosion of numerous and diverse techniques for achieving the subjugation of bodies and the control of populations' (Foucault 1984: 140). As Foucault (1991: 194) writes emphatically,

We must cease once and for all to describe the effects of power in negative terms: "it excludes", it "represses", it "censors", it "abstracts", it
"masks", it "conceals". In fact, power produces; it produces reality; it
produces domains of objects and rituals of truth.

This perspective illuminates the productiveness of biopower, where biopower can be used 'to designate what brought life and its mechanisms into
the realm of explicit calculations and made knowledge-power an agent of
transformation of human life' (Foucault 1984: 143).

Secondly, whilst disciplinary power can be characterized as making
'docile bodies', these are not bodies at the total mercy of a sovereign form
of power. Modern forms of power function in terms of *relations of power*,
an emphasis that rebukes views of 'fundamental power. It is to give oneself
as the object of analysis power relations and not power itself' (Foucault
1983: 219). Summing up this relationship, Foucault (1983: 219) explains
that '[a]t the very heart of the power relationship, and constantly provoking it, are the recalcitrance of will and the intransigence of freedom'. For
Foucault (1983: 220), 'power is produced from one moment to the next'.
For this reason Foucault (1984: 93) can argue '[p]ower is everywhere; not
because it embraces everything, but because it comes from everywhere'.
Disciplinary power works via individuals disciplining themselves, it is a
form of surveillance that is internalized (Foucault 1991). It is not a power
that forces by sheer violence.

In asserting and reasserting this relational emphasis, Foucault is making
an important distinction from top-down, hierarchized forms of power, of
which sovereign power typifies. It is instructive to recognize why Foucault
sought to examine and elucidate these relations of power. In response to
questions pertaining to his work on power, Foucault (1983: 209) exclaims
'it is not power, but the subject, which is the general theme of my work'.
Thus Foucault needed to study the workings of *power* in order to consider
the problem of the *subject*. In a similar fashion, the biopedagogies of the
obesity epidemic can be used to analyze how relations of power influence
the formation of the contemporary healthy subject.

Integral to the analysis of power and as a consequence, the subject,
was the recognition of what Foucault terms the influence of the 'norm',
the *normalizing society*. For Dreyfus and Rabinow (1983: 258), the relation of biopower to normalizing practices lies in the former being able to
'define the normal in advance and then proceed to isolate and deal with
the anomalies given that definition'. Similarly, Anna Laura Stoler (2000:
83) observes the import Foucault attached to analysing 'the norm that circulates between the processes of disciplining and regularization and that
articulates the individual and the population'. Normalizing mechanisms
are evident in biopedagogies of obesity that delineate normal body weight
and shape, and via those acts that segregate and manage individuals.
Indeed, the work in this volume points to the importance of appreciating

the extent to which new norms are being configured via the biopedagogies of obesity.

Biopower thus forms an important angle from which to analyse the constitution of subjects (and consequently, processes of normalization). The shift to a mode of biopower mode displaces a focus on 'humans needs . . . as ends in themselves or as subjects of a philosophic discourse which sought to discover their essential nature' (Dreyfus and Rabinow 1983: 139–40). Under the sway of biopower, human needs are seen 'instrumentally and empirically, as the means for the increase of the state's power. Foucault thus demonstrates the relationship between the new administrative concept of human welfare and the growth of bio-power' (Dreyfus and Rabinow 1983: 139–40). Biopower sheds light on the problem of the subject because it shows up the control of individuals and populations through *bios* practices associated with the body in the modern state. There are however dilemmas to attend to that pertain, as Rabinow and Rose (2006) point out, to extending Foucault's analysis from the twentieth century into the twenty-first.

Foucault's (1965; 1975; 1976; 1984; 1991) examination of the human sciences, medicine, psychology and psychiatry, and criminality provide interrogations of the norm, and the relationship of normalisation to the constitution of the subject. In these studies where Foucault used his innovative approach to the analysis of historical material, it can be argued that '[t]he new political rationality of bio-power was therefore connected with the nascent empirical human sciences' (Dreyfus and Rabinow 1983: 137). There is a difference to be considered between the contemporary twentieth century at the time of Foucault's writing and our contemporary twenty-first century (Rabinow and Rose 2006). This is an important distinction. Foucault's research by his own designation, began with a problem in the present, a point accentuated in his discussion of genealogy (Foucault 1977).[4] The contemporary concerns that prompted Foucault's work differ in some respects to ours, and more obviously, empirical sciences in our contemporary context cannot be considered 'nascent' in the same way they were at the time of emergence of biopower. There are now well-established human sciences, and there are those that are nascent, one could argue, via their increasing specificity. The rise of genomic medicine is a case in point (Rabinow and Rose 2006). Reflecting on biopower and these up-and-coming sciences, Rabinow and Rose pose the question as to whether we are 'in an emergent moment of vital politics' (2006: 215). What follows is their suggestion of the value of biopower.

> The concept of biopower, used in a precise fashion, related to empirical investigations and subject to inventive development, would surely take its place as a key part in an analytical toolkit adequate to the diagnosis of what Gilles Deleuze has termed "the near future".
>
> (Rabinow and Rose 2006: 215)

Critical analysis of notions of the obesity epidemic is one empirical investigation that can contribute to this task of examining a possible emergent moment of 'vital politics'.

BIOPOWER AND BIOPEDAGOGIES

A striking feature of the obesity epidemic is the way in which public discourses have become integral to the promulgation of knowledge about the 'problem of obesity' (Gard and Wright 2005). Whilst health clinics and classrooms may appear the commonsense sites where pedagogies pertaining to obesity are to be struck, these sites represent only a fraction of the spaces where this pedagogy occurs. Pedagogy, then, needs to be understood more broadly as a complex and relational cultural practice through which knowledge is produced (Lusted 1986; McWilliam 1996; Tyler 2004). Although the term pedagogy traditionally implies a school context, as McWilliam (1996) argues, it is also theorized as a practice in the social sciences, humanities and the visual and performing arts. Here the interrogation of sites of communication and knowledge exchange beyond the classroom have generated lively debates in the ways of understanding the pedagogical relationship (Gallop 1995; Gore 1998 2002; McWilliam and Tyler 1996). As Henry Giroux (1999) argues, pedagogy can no longer be confined to the site of schooling, using the term 'public pedagogy', he suggests it needs to be understood as applying to political sites in 'which identities are shaped, desires mobilized, and experiences take on form and meaning'.

These elusive yet provocative descriptions of pedagogy prompt a reconsideration of how meaning is formed and disseminated. Biopedagogies occur in myriad political sites involved in the construction of identities that instruct and form meaning. Biopedagogy then, is the art and practice of teaching of 'life', of *bios* in this 'biopower mode'. Attention to life in terms of biopower's two poles demands a pedagogical concern with both the individualized body and with the species (the population). Biopedagogies are practices that impart knowledge writ large, occurring at multiple levels across countless domains and sites. As a concept biopedagogy offers to accomplish two important tasks; it draws attention to the pedagogical practices inhering in the biopolitical (for example, public health promotion) and secondly, it offers a means to formulate an empirical analytic to interrogate the concealed pedagogical practices of biopower.

Given this intimate connection between biopedagogy and biopolitics, the question needs to be posed, what is the biopolitical, or more exactly, what are its characteristics? Foucault provides three points to note regarding biopolitics in the final of 1975–76 Lectures. The first is that biopolitics is 'not dealing with the individual-as-body. It is a new body, a multiple body . . . [b]iopolitics deals with the population, with the population as political problem' (Foucault 2003: 245). The second point concerns the nature of the phenomena, the population and its unpredictability. In Foucault's words 'the phenomena addressed by biopolitics are, essentially, aleatory events that occur within a population that exists over a period of time' (Foucault 2003: 246). In the third point Foucault suggests how regularizing practices may function. Biopolitics 'will introduce mechanisms with a certain number of functions that are very different from the function of disciplinary mechanisms' (Foucault 2003: 246).

> The mechanisms introduced by biopolitics include forecasts, statistical estimates, and overall measures. And their purpose is not to modify any given phenomenon as such, or to modify a given individual insofar as he is an individual, but, essentially, to intervene at the level at which these general phenomena are determined, to intervene a the level of their generality. The mortality rate has to modified or lowered; life expectancy has to be increased; the birth rate has to be stimulated. And most important of all, regulatory mechanisms must be established to establish an equilibrium, maintain an average, establish a sort of homeostasis, and compensate for variations within this general population and its aleatory field.
>
> (Foucault 2003: 246)

In the biopolitical mode, biopedagogies, function to affect populations, they are concerned with the aleatorical nature of 'population', and they target concerns of life such as birth rate, or obesity. In so doing, their function is to impart knowledges that make meaning, and are attached to the shaping of identities and desires of life.

However, considering that Foucault depicted that there were two poles of biopower, what of disciplinary power and biopedagogies? Given Foucault's description of the two powers dovetailing together, how are we to envisage the relationship between a biopower that is disciplinary and the biopolitical biopower that regularizes? I suggest that some clues to this question can be drawn from Rabinow and Rose (2006) who present biopower as a 'plane of actuality' that comprises three elements (they suggest this is a minimum). In summary these pertain firstly to the promulgation of certain *truths about 'life'* that are '[k]nowledge of vital life processes' (Rabinow and Rose 2006: 215). Secondly, there is need to consider the effects of *power over 'life'*, 'power relations that take living beings as their object' (Rabinow and Rose 2006: 215). Thirdly, there is the question of the effect of *subjectification on 'life'*, 'modes of subjectification through which subjects work on themselves qua living beings—as well as their multiple combinations' (Rabinow and Rose 2006: 215).[5] An extensive quotation is provided below:

- One or more truth discourses about the 'vital' character of living human beings, and an array of authorities considered competent to tell the truth.
- Strategies for intervention upon collective existence in the name of life and health, initially addressed to populations that may or may not be territorialized upon the nation, society or pre-given communities, but may also be specified in terms of emergent biosocial collectivities, sometimes specified in terms of categories of race, ethnicity, gender or religion, as in the emerging forms of genetic or biological citizenship.
- Modes of subjectification, through which individuals are brought to work on themselves, under certain forms of authority, in relation to truth discourses, by means of practices of the self, in the name of their own life and health, that of their family or some other collectivity, or indeed in the name of the life or health of the population as a whole.

(Rabinow and Rose 2006: 197)

These elements hold out promise when pedagogy is taken as a cultural practice that imparts knowledge concerning life and is a cultural practice through 'which identities are shaped, desires mobilized, and experiences take on form and meaning' (Giroux, 1999). Consideration of the workings of truth, power and modes of subjectification thus take shape as analytic tools for interrogating biopower's pedagogies of life.

BIOPEDAGOGIES OF LIFE

I now turn to sketch out some possible ways that the above elements may be drawn on to engage an analysis of biopedagogies that can contribute to the task of interrogating what Rabinow and Rose (2006) call an 'emergent moment of vital politics'. It is also essential to contemplate both disciplinary and regularizing techniques of power, that is, the influence of biopedagogies as both individualizing and massifying. However, to ascribe or catalogue these under the umbrella of one of these elements may be to miss the subtle point of how these elements works together. As I have stated elsewhere (Harwood 2006), truth, power and subjectification are each intimately associated with the other. As such, an analysis needs to take into consideration both how to identify these elements and how to be aware of their inter-relatedness. Having made this point, I want to stress that modes of subjectification are crucial to an analysis of biopower and specifically, biopedagogies. Modes of subjectification are a key point from which to grasp how subjection operates in biopower. I begin by discussing each of the elements, then move to elucidate what modes of subjectification offer an analysis of biopower and biopedagogy.

Considering truth discourses about the vital character of living beings demands attention be paid to biopedagogical knowledge. If discourses of life that shape identity are communicated in a biopedagogical relation, we need to ask what are the instructions that are being given? Who are the 'authorities' that give the instructions, or more precisely, who are the pedagogues? In a given moment, at a given point in the struggles for life in the biopower mode, what are the biopedagogies of truth, and who tells them? At the core of their urgency is the impetus of ensuring 'life'. Biopedagogical discourses such as those of the 'obesity discourse' increasingly identify children as a 'risk' population. Instruction is disseminated about food types, food intake, body shapes, and a generalized message is promulgated that instructs the population that it is unhealthy if too many of its numbers are obese. At a micro level, teachers and others can direct and discipline individuals regarding true discourses, acting as pedagogues in an individualising and disciplinary process. Pollock (2003: 248) notes this effect with reproductive endocrinologists, who can 'be understood . . . to be the administrators of the bodies in the clinics in a way very different from the sovereign'.

The second of the three elements is characterized by Rabinow and Rose (2006: 215) as 'strategies', these are the 'power relations that take living beings as their object'. Questions can be posed as to what strategies are in place to ensure that living beings can indeed become objects to be worked on, to be pedagogized. It is relevant to note that while Rabinow and Rose (2006) appear to distinguish the authority to speak the truth from relations of power strategies (perhaps for the purpose of their outline), the two are interconnected (Harwood 2006). Following this reasoning, it could be asked, what power relations make the strategies of speaking the truth possible? What relations of power make the pedagogue? Schools are an exemplar of one of the targets for the strategies of power geared towards getting the population's children more active, 'thin' or changing their eating patterns. In a disciplinary mode, biopedagogies place individuals in schools under constant surveillance, whilst its regularizing techniques instruct the population on the risks its children pose to the health of the nation.

Modes of subjectification, the third element, brings attention to the role of the subject in the vital practices of life. This analytic approach involves how 'subjects work on themselves qua living beings' (Rabinow and Rose 2006: 215). Reflecting the focus of the later years of Foucault's work, subjectification takes up the concern of the subject. Displacing any assumption of the subject as an object to be acted on, subjectification situates the subject in active fashion, as fundamental to the process of becoming a subject. Succinctly, the distinction lies in the emphasis placed on the subject as *active* in its own constitution (it is not merely acted *upon*). Thus the emphasis is on 'how the individual constitutes him or herself through a process of subjectification' (Lacombe 1996: 341). The observation by Holmes et al. (2006) of the emphasis placed on being 'an active and responsible citizen who will not be a burden on the health care system' is a case in point.[6] The patient is thus the recipient of a biopedagogy that inculcates them into a complex web that is far more than 'health' in a rudimentary sense; their interaction with the biopedagogy and their self-discipline are intimately connected with the good of the population: the biopolitics of bios. This attention to modes of subjectification can explicitly draw out the effects of 'norms', as Pollock's (2003) research with egg donors attests. Reflecting on her interviews, she writes '[t]he donors I spoke with generally accepted the norms that the clinic put forth and were not troubled by the questions unless they made them look bad' (Pollock 2003: 252).

Modes of subjectification are accordingly a decisive component for the analysis of biopower, and by consequence, the examination of biopedagogies. This is because subjectification is integral to processes of subjection. Biopedagogies influence the modes of subjectification by pressing the population to monitor themselves, often through intensifying knowledge on 'obesity' related risks/issues, and 'instructing' them on how to eat healthily, and stay active.

How are these modes to be analysed? There are some clues to be found in Foucault's work. Here I refer to his lecture on 10 March 1982, part of the 1981–82 lectures on the *Hermeneutic of Subject*, at the Collège de France (Foucault 2005). In a discussion of parrhesia, Foucault (2005: 371) makes this observation of the disciple's self-work in relation to 'the communication of these true discourses, of communication between the person who delivers them and the person who receives them and constructs from them an equipment for life'.[7] In this quote can be seen an accent on the subject's role in 'receiving them', and in how they are incorporated into life. Whilst this analysis of pre-Christian practices can't be taken as analogous to contemporary practices, there are nonetheless related points to consider, principally, that the subject is actively involved.[8] So we can ask how or by what techniques did such a subject receive and construct these true discourses in a practice of subjectification?

> So a technique and an ethics of silence, a technique and an ethics of listening, and a technique and an ethics also of reading and writing, which are so many exercises for the subjectivation of true discourse.
>
> (Foucault 2005: 372)

In this relation, the disciple is presented with the master's true discourse. The subjectification of this true discourse, as a practice of the self is accomplished via techniques of silence, of listening, of reading and of writing. Foucault's account of pagan modes of the subjectification of a true discourse offer an emphasis on the role of the subject, the micropractices in the constitution of the self. These practices speak to more than *resistance*. Attending to this example prompts us to reflect more cogently on relations of power in the biopower mode.

Taking the above example as a cue, what can be drawn, or more exactly, what exercise/s may the contemporary twenty-first century subject use in the subjectification of the true discourses of biopedagogy? This places into relief the other two elements, the truth about vital life and relations of power. In regard to the latter, we can ask: how are such exercises influenced by relations of power? What strategies are at work? To this can be added questions that pertain to the two poles of biopower: What disciplinary techniques are used on the individual that individualize him or her, and what exercises do these provoke? What techniques of regularization used on the population affect the subjectification of true discourses? How are these to be understood at the level of the population, at the level of the individual?

CONCLUSION

Biopedagogies have a central function in contemporary biopower via their contribution to the task of regularising aleatory populations, and in the disciplining of the individual. Yet what is to be made of the all-important question of change, transformation, struggle, or to frame this in the well-known Foucauldian term, 'resistance'? Isn't the task of analysis to take in the struggles that inhere in life, at its many levels, and not simply portray a prism of seemingly static 'things as they are'. Further, doesn't it behold us to attempt to think differently such that there is always the possibility of other possibilities?

In their valuable work *Michel Foucault, Beyond Structuralism and Hermeneutics* Hubert Dreyfus and Paul Rabinow (1983) pose the question of biopower and resistance. A question that I maintain needs to be at the forefront of analysis of biopower, and certainly, biopedagogies. They ask,

> How is resistance to biopower to be strengthened? Dialectical arguments which appeal to the correct theoretical understanding of human beings and society are hardly sufficient to move large numbers of people and, following Foucault's analysis, are part of the current problem. Clearly the rhetorical dimension is crucial here. Granted that the Platonic conception of truth is "our longest lie," must we be reduced to a Platonic conception of rhetorical or pragmatic discourse as mere manipulation? Or is there an art of interpretation which draws on other resources and opens up the possibility of using discourse to oppose domination?
>
> (Dreyfus and Rabinow 1983: 206–7)

My response to this question is to reiterate the significance of attending to the modes of subjectification. These are I argue, the points at which, to loosely quote these authors, to 'open up possibilities of using discourse to oppose domination'. Modes of subjectification offer alternative accounts of the truths of regularizing discourses. We need to ask, does everyone believe what they are told? And importantly, what are the risks our research runs of assuming so? When an individual does believe them, what exercise/s are accomplished in the subjectification of the true discourse? This point highlights the importance of subjugated knowledges, and their possible insurrectionary potential (Harwood and Rasmussen 2007).

Modes of subjectification draw attention to the relational condition of biopower. This is a distinction from the work of Agamben (1998; 2000) and works that draw on his interpretation of biopower such as Lewis (2006). As such, attention to the modes of subjectification call into question appraisals of 'bare life' where the subject is situated outside, where there is the danger of conceptualising the subject as both unable to resist, nor involved in their own subjection.[9] With regard to the debate between Agamben's reading of biopower and that of Foucault's (Dillon 2005; Genel 2006; Margaroni 2005; Ojakangas 2005), attention to the modes of subjectification may contribute a perspective on the relationship between contemporary juridico-legal power and biopolitics on the one hand, and sovereign power and the biopower on the other. Practically, this may comprise empirical research with those whom, following Agamben, are 'bare life' or in a 'state of exception'. Such work would explicitly endeavour to analyse the modes of subjectification of true discourses of the state by such individuals. While acknowledging the difficulty of access (if it is at all possible), it nevertheless behoves contemplation or else risks relegating social theory research to its own state of exception, calling into question the productiveness of our activities.

Then there is the norm. Ojakangas (2005) cites François Ewald's (1992: 173) point that '[t]he norm or normative space, knows no outside . . . the norm integrates anything which might attempt to go beyond it—nothing, nobody, whatever difference it might display, can ever claim to be exterior'. As Ojakangas (2005: 16) argues, '[i]n the case of the norm, these exceptions are not however, taken out (*ex-capere*), but taken in (*in-capere*)'. Analysis of the modes of subjectification to a true discourse (such as the biopedagogical) accentuates the force of normalization in contemporary society. Lastly, modes of subjection bring to the fore the aleatory quality of the population. A quality that is, perhaps, our most genius ally in any resistance to the homogenizing attempts of biopower to regulate and discipline the populace.

NOTES

1. There is an alternative construal of biopower used by Giorgio Agamben (1998; 2000) and by Antonio Negri (Hardt and Negri 2000). This work, as Rabinow and Rose address in their germane paper is 'misleading' in its elucidation and application of biopower. The crux of their critique is disagreement with an interpretation of biopower that focuses on death.

2. Care needs to be taken here that the assumption isn't made that biopower 'cleanly' replaces all forms of sovereign power (juridico-legal power). See the 1975–76 Lectures where Foucault discusses 'Nazi society' (Foucault 2003). See also Judith Butler (2004), and Rasmussen and Harwood (2009).
3. Rabinow and Dreyfus (1983) and Rabinow and Rose (2006) put these poles in an inverse order. Here I follow Foucault's (1984) order from *The History of Sexuality Volume 1, An Introduction.*
4. The emergence of each pole of biopower is situated historically, commencing in the seventeenth century and noting their effects in the eighteenth century and nineteenth century (Foucault, 1984) and in the final of the 1975–76 Lectures, the twentieth century (Foucault, 2003).
5. Here Rabinow and Rose (2006) use the word subjectification, which is used throughout this chapter. Elsewhere (and in translations of Foucault) the word subjectivation is used. Lacombe (1996: 350) explains that 'Foucault uses the French word subjectivation which is translated as either "subjectification" or "subjectivization"'.
6. See also Perron et al. (2004) for a diagrammatic depiction of 'bio-power indicators'.
7. For a discussion on parrhesia and truth telling in relation to sexuality see Harwood (2004).
8. A difference is noted by Foucault (2005: 333) between objectification of oneself, what he describes as a Christian ascesis of self renunciation 'whose essential moment is, the objectification of the self in a true discourse' and a pagan ascesis, which 'involves coming together with oneself, the essential moment of which is not the objectification of the self in a true discourse, but the subjectivation of a true discourse in a practice and exercise of oneself on oneself'.
9. While there are compelling arguments for the use of Agamben's concept of bare life to situate contemporary political practices such as the internment of prisoners in Guantanamo Bay, my point here is to dispute recourse to bare life as an underlying principle of biopower. This is a point addressed by Oja-kangas (2005).

REFERENCES

Agamben, G. (1998) *Home Sacer: Sovereign Power and Bare Life*, Stanford, California: Stanford University Press.
———.(2000) *Remnants of Auschwitz: The Witness and the Archive*, New York: Zone Books.
Butler, J. (2004) *Precarious Life: The Powers of Mourning and Violence*, London: Verso.
Dillon, M. (2005) 'Cared to death: the biopoliticised time of your life', *Foucault Studies*, 2: 37–46.
Dreyfus, H.L. and Rabinow, P. (1983) *Michel Foucault: Beyond Structuralism and Hermeneutics*, New York: Harvester Wheatsheaf.
Ewald, F. (1992) 'A Power Without an Exterior', in T.J. Armstrong (ed.) *Michel Foucault: Philosopher*, New York: Harvester Wheatsheaf.
Foucault, M. (1965) *Madness and Civilisation: A History of Insanity in the Age of Reason*, New York: Pantheon.
———.(1975) *The Birth of the Clinic*, New York: Vintage.
———.(1976) *Mental Illness and Psychology*, New York: Harper Collins.

———.(1977) 'Nietzsche, Genealogy, History', in D.F. Bouchard (ed.) *Language, Counter-Memory, Practice: Selected Essays and Interviews*, Ithaca, New York: Cornell University Press.

———.(1983) 'The Subject and Power', in H.L. Dreyfus and P. Rabinow (eds) *Michel Foucault: Beyond Structuralism and Hermeneutics*, 2nd ed., University of Chicago: University of Chicago press.

———.(1984) *The History of Sexuality, Volume I: An Introduction*, Harmondsworth, Middlesex, England: Peregrine, Penguin Books.

———.(1991) *Discipline and Punish: The Birth of the Prison*, London: Penguin Books.

———.(2000) 'Truth and Power', in J.D. Faubion (ed.) *Power, The Essential Works of Michel Foucault*, Vol. III, New York: The New Press.

———.(2003) *Society Must Be Defended: Lectures at the Collège De France 1975–76*, New York: Picador.

———.(2005) *The Hermeneutics of the Subject: Lectures at the Collège De France 1981–82*, trans. G. Burchell, New York: Palgrave Macmillan.

Gallop, J. (ed.) (1995) *Pedagogy: The Question of Impersonation*, Indiana: University of Bloomington Press.

Gard, M. and Wright, J. (2005) *The Obesity Epidemic: Science, Morality and Ideology*, Oxford: Routledge.

Gastaldo, D. (1997) 'Is Health Education Good for You? Rethinking Health education through the concept of bio-power', in A. Peterson and R. Bunton (eds) *Foucault, Health and Medicine*, London: Routledge.

Genel, K. (2006) 'The Question of Biopower: Foucault and Agamben', *Rethinking Marxism*, 18(1): 43–62.

Giroux, H. (1999) *Cultural Studies as Public Pedagogy: making the pedagogical more political*, retrieved 15 February 2005, from www.vusst.hr/ENCLOPAEDIA/main.htm

Gore, J.M. (1998) 'Disciplining Bodies: On the Continuity of Power Relations in Pedagogy', in T.S. Popkewitz and M. Brennan (eds) *Foucault's Challenge: Discourse, Knowledge, and Power in Education*, New York: Teacher's College Press.

———.(2002) 'Micro-Level Techniques of Power in the Pedagogical Production of Class, Race, Gender and Other Relations', in H.S. Shapiro and S. Shapiro (eds) *Body Movements: Pedagogy, Politics and Social Change*, New Jersey: Hampton Press.

Hardt, M. and Negri, A. (2000) *Empire*, Cambridge, MA: Harvard University Press.

Harwood, V. (2004) 'Telling truths: wounded truths and the activity of truth telling', *Discourse: studies in the cultural politics of education*, 25(4): 467–76.

———. (2006) *Diagnosing 'Disorderly' Children: A Critique of Behaviour Disorder Discourses*, London: Routledge.

Harwood, V. and Rasmussen, M.L. (2007) 'Scrutinizing sexuality and psychopathology: a Foucauldian inspired strategy for qualitative data analysis', *International Journal of Qualitative Studies in Education*, 20(1): 31–50.

Holmes, D., Perron, A.M. and Savoi, M. (2006) 'Governing therapy choices: power/knowledge in the treatment of progressive renal failure', *Philosophy, Ethics, and Humanities in Medicine*,1(12): retrieved 20 January 2006, from http://www.peh-med.com/content/1/1/12

Hook, D. (2003) 'Analogues of power: reading psychotherapy through the sovereignty-discipline-government complex', *Theory and Psychology*, 13(5): 605–28.

Lacombe, D. (1996) 'Reforming Foucault: a critique of the social control thesis', *The British Journal of Sociology*, 47(2): 332–52.

Lewis, T.E. (2006) 'The school as an exceptional space: rethinking education from the perspective of the biopedagogical', *Educational Theory*, 56(2): 159–76.

Lusted, D. (1986) 'Why pedagogy', *Screen*, 27(5): 2–15.

Margaroni, M. (2005) 'Care and abandonment: a response to Mike Ojakangas' 'Impossible dialogue on bio-power: Agamben and Foucault', *Foucault Studies*, 2: 29–36.

McWilliam, E. (1996) 'Pedagogies, technologies and bodies', in E. McWilliam and P.G. Taylor (eds) *Pedagogy, Technology and the Body*, New York: Peter Lang.

McWilliam, E. and Tyler, D. (eds) (1996) *Pedagogy, Technology and the Body*, New York: Peter Lang.

Ojakangas, M. (2005) 'Impossible dialogue: Agamben and Foucault', *Foucault Studies*, 2: 5–28.

Perron, A.M., Fluet, C. and Holmes, D. (2004) 'Agents of care and agents of the state: bio-power and nursing practice', *Journal of Advanced Nursing*, 50(5): 536–44.

Pollock, A. (2003) 'Complicating power in high-tech reproduction: narratives of anonymous paid egg donors', *Journal of Medical Humanities*, 24(3/4): 241–63.

Rabinow, P. and Rose, N. (2006) 'Biopower today', *Biosocieties*, 1(2): 195–217.

Rasmussen, M.L. and Harwood, V. (2009) 'Young people, education and unlawful citizenship: spectral sovereignty and governmentality in Australia', *Globalisation, Societies and Education*, 7(1): (forthcoming).

Rose, N. (2006) *The Politics of Life Itself: Biomedicine, Power and Subjectivity in the Twenty-First Century*, Princeton, NJ: Princeton University Press.

Stoler, A.L. (2000) *Race and the Education of Desire, Foucault's History of Sexuality and the Colonial Order of Things*, Durham and London: Duke University Press.

Tyler, W. (2004). 'Silent, invisible, total: pedagogic discourse and the age of information', in J. Muller, B. Davies and A. Morais (eds) *Reading Bernstein, Researching Bernstein*, London: Routledge/Falmer.

3   Friends, Enemies and the Cultural Politics of Critical Obesity Research

Michael Gard

At least as far back as the publication of Ulrich Beck's (1992) *Risk Society*, social commentators have contemplated the idea that late capitalism might become a game not of accumulating goods but avoiding 'bads'. Beck's original thesis proposed that the modern world produced new kinds of risks that were changing the nature of global politics and forging new local and global alliances. Modern risks were different because they were too big to be contained within the borders of nation states (think nuclear disasters) and because they were the fruits of 'progress' (think ecological destruction). Perhaps most important of all, modern risks were different because their scale made them impossible to insure against; no amount of money could undo the damage of an environmental catastrophe. It is this final difference that Beck saw as providing the kinetic energy for social transformation. Beck's ideas drew a predictable chorus of critics, partly due to their sheer ambition, but equally because of his later links with New Labour's 'Third Way' social agenda in the UK.

And yet as time goes by, Beck's critics might wonder about the wisdom of judging him by the company he kept. His assessment was that new global and local alliances and new forms of capitalism would emerge as risk management began to compete with the exploitation of opportunity as a key financial calculus. Recent international deliberations about mechanisms for dealing with climate change (such as those concerning international carbon trading schemes or plans for dealing with environmental refugees) look to me like as precise a vindication of *Risk Society*'s central ideas as we could hope to see.

More recently, the prominent sociologist Frank Furedi has also placed risk avoidance at the centre of modern Western culture in a series of influential publications, most notably his 1997 work *Culture of Fear: risk taking and the morality of low expectation* (revised editions have appeared in 2002 and 2005). Furedi argues that Western culture has lost its nerve. It no longer believes in its capacity for 'progress' and always asks 'what are the risks?' before it asks 'what are the possibilities?'. His culprits are a large and diverse group: social conservatives, environmentalists, sensationalist media and impoverished political leadership to name a few amongst many others.

I became interested in Furedi's work because of his interest in obesity. I noticed that despite the apparent absence of any sustained scholarship on the subject of his own, Furedi was prepared to pronounce that talk of an 'obesity crisis' was not only unfounded but also an example of 'fear culture' in action. This may seem an uncharitable reaction, but it did strike me as odd that such a prominent academic might choose to believe the account of a small number of 'obesity sceptics'. The impression I gained from reading his work and listening to his public lectures was that he had simply pounced opportunistically on the work of 'obesity sceptics' because it suited his own theoretical leanings.

What follows in this chapter is a somewhat anecdotal account of my experiences as one of a small international group of 'obesity sceptics'—some of whom are contributors to this volume—and what we might call the cultural politics of critical obesity research. My purpose is threefold: first, to interrogate some of the complacent alliances that form between 'like minds' in critical obesity research; second, to explore some of the intellectual resources that have yet to be harnessed by critical obesity researchers and; third, to contribute to scholarship about the cultural significance of 'obesity epidemic' discourse.

While its personal flavour may worry some readers, my aspiration here is conventionally academic: to illuminate by trying to connect and disconnect ideas. Throughout, Beck's warning that risk undermines traditional political and theoretical alliances will be a mostly unstated presence. Above all, though, I want to show that, as with the example of Frank Furedi, what matters in the world—but particularly the world of obesity science—is belief, not truth, and that this is a 'truth' critical obesity scholars might profitably exploit in their own work. Our job as dissenting voices may be less about establishing the truth about obesity but rather exploiting people's beliefs.

ON NOT BEING TALKED ABOUT

The work of scholars who for the purposes of this chapter I will call the 'obesity sceptics' has largely been ignored in the medico-scientific literature. A few dissenting articles have appeared in significant international journals (for example Campos, Saguy, Ernsberger, Oliver and Gaesser 2006) although these have had little if any impact on mainstream scientific and popular 'obesity crisis' discourse. In fact, 'obesity epidemic' sceptics have been so completely ignored that national health authorities and high profile medical researchers continue to claim, for example, that obesity is as big a problem as global warming (CBS News 2006). The durability and popularity of the idea that, *à la* global warming, obesity could wreak catastrophic damage on human civilization as we know it is surely compelling evidence of the absence of a widely circulating counterbalancing discourse.

The publication of *The Obesity Epidemic: science, morality and ideology* (Gard and Wright 2005) received a steady trickle of mainstream and alternative print and electronic media interest following its publication in 2005, particularly on the libertarian online magazine *Spiked*. In 2006 I received an invitation to appear on *Counterpoint*, an Australian radio program hosted by Michael Duffy, widely seen as a conservative member of the national commentariat although he is also probably more accurately pigeon-holed as a free-market libertarian. I appeared on *Counterpoint* not long after Frank Furedi. Furedi, a regular writer for *Spiked*, has been interviewed a number of times for Duffy's show and his books are mentioned frequently for reasons that are worth dwelling on.

One of Furedi's (1997) central arguments is that a preoccupation with risk and fear robs Western culture of its ability to confront confidently the challenges it *does* face and fatally undermines the idea of progress. A generation of poststructuralist, feminist and environmentally minded scholars have argued that the idea of 'progress' was one of the first ideological casualties of post 1960s deconstructionist, feminist and queer social theory and post 1970s green politics. In other words, 'progress' became a highly problematic term within leftist political circles and has been an important 'culture wars' battleground. Furedi is certainly no friend of cultural conservatives but his attempts to resuscitate 'progress' make him potentially useful to enemies of the left.

This situation should not be unfamiliar. Many authors in this volume reference Foucauldian, feminist and poststructuralist inspired scholars such as Lupton whose work on 'medicalization' draws critical attention to the legitimization of ever expanding governmental intervention in people's lives in the name of 'health'. This is an interesting development because the kind of obesity scepticism presented in this volume emanates from university based social science scholarship, a field of endeavour generally associated with social democratic ideals in which governments *are expected* to intervene in people's lives. For example, there are relatively few university-based social scientists or feminists who argue in favour of unfettered small government capitalism in areas of public policy such as school education, prisons, the environment or health. And yet the critique of 'medicalization' finds scholars from the traditionally leftist social sciences questioning one of the most obvious forms of modern government oversight. We should not forget that there are those who argue for a war on obesity precisely on socially democratic/progressive grounds (for example, Critser 2000 and 2003).

What is at stake here is the aged question of whether we create a better society by allowing people to express their desires freely or by forcing them to keep their desires in check. For libertarians like Furedi and Michael Duffy society needs, first, more faith in people's ability to make sound choices for themselves, second, less government intervention in our lives and, third, less moral opprobrium directed at what we eat and how we look.

As a critical obesity scholar, there are parts of this ideological package that are appealing to me and parts that are not. During our interview, Duffy seemed predictably enthusiastic about my misgivings of creeping medical surveillance of people's, particularly children's, body weight. But as a determined social constructionist I had to challenge what I assumed to be his free-market libertarian bias: no, I did not think it was enough to say simply that people should be allowed to eat what they want. From my perspective, it is very difficult to speak of pre-given human desires that both precede culture and provide a reliable moral or dietary compass. Desires, I assume, are *acquired*; they are a product of prevailing social conditions, not a cure for them. Amongst other things, this means that Western diets *are* significantly shaped by the imperatives of global capital. And although there are nutritionists who argue that human brains are 'hard wired' to crave sugar, fat and salt, there is no convincing evidence that the amount of sugar, fat and salt in modern fast and convenience foods is anything other than the product of successful marketing and the global over-production of these substances. Should we, for example, be unconcerned that fast food multinational companies target poorer communities in order to sell more low-quality food?

I cannot be sure what Frank Furedi thinks about food, but my guess is that he believes we should worry less about how food is made, marketed and sold and simply leave parents to monitor what children eat as they see fit. Indeed, he argues strongly that the world has too many 'experts' on parenting, to the point that many parents think they need—and actively seek out—experts to tell them how to parent.

These potential areas of disagreement aside, Duffy hosts a stimulating and thought provoking show that often presents conservative ideas at their most sophisticated. However, *The Obesity Epidemic* (Gard and Wright 2005) also found an audience in less intellectually minded conservative circles. For example, the right wing web site *Political Correctness Watch* (2005) (subtitled 'The creeping dictatorship of the left') praised the book because, the site argued, it offered arguments against 'nanny-state' leftists who wanted to tell the rest of us how to live (jonjayray 2005). Actually, there are a number of elements to this argument. For this form of hard right thinking, 'nanny-state' politics is not only hyper-interventionist and power hungry, it is also anti-pleasure. Ergo, if Gard and Wright are saying there is no obesity crisis then there is no reason for health authorities to intrude on my capacity to consume what I want to consume.

In passing it is worth emphasising the ideological intensity that is tied up in terms such as 'nanny-state' when used in the United States. For example, the Harvard University researcher Kelly Brownell was widely criticized and ridiculed in conservative circles when he campaigned to raise taxes on junk food and subsidize the cost of fruit and vegetables. For many of his critics, Brownell's ideas were simply un-American. Similarly, Eric Schlosser (2001), the author of *Fast Food Nation: what the all-American meal is doing to the world*, was the target of sustained and orchestrated media vilification because of his criticisms of the fast food multinationals (for an example of press coverage of this, see Burkeman 2006). As it happens, *The Obesity Epidemic* used and praised Schlosser's book, and yet *Political Correctness Watch* scored Schlosser bad, Gard and Wright good.

But in a striking and even perverse parallel, *The Obesity Epidemic* was also featured on the web sites of a number of fat acceptance groups. This is striking because, in many ways, fat acceptance represents a constituency that is diametrically opposed to the positions taken by the likes of *Political Correctness Watch*. On the one hand, fat acceptance groups argue that we need to legislate in order to reduce discrimination against fat people (some even suggest fines and jail sentences for people found guilty of discrimination), that fat people are not morally responsible for their fatness (they argue that fat people are usually the victims of biology) and that social infrastructure be modified in order to make it easier for fat people to participate more fully in society (for example, they argue for bigger seats on aircraft and wider turnstiles in train stations). On the other hand, anti-'nanny-state' groups like *Political Correctness Watch* are vehemently opposed to the influence of 'minority' interests, fiercely reject the idea that we should legislate in their favour, and bemoan 'litigation culture' which they see as undermining personal responsibility. Indeed, some right wing authors have gone out of their way to accuse fat acceptance activists of encouraging and contributing to the breakdown of important social norms, as well as being in a simple state of self-denial concerning the individual responsibility of fat people for their weight (for a virulent example, see Fumento 1997).

Putting to one side the apparently inevitable meanness and bigotry of hard right rhetoric, I have some sympathy for these views. In particular, the consistent argument put forward by fat acceptance groups that most fat people do not eat any more than people who are not fat is extremely dubious. For example, in her forward for the 1983 volume *Shadow on a Tightrope: writings by women on fat oppression*, Vivian F. Mayer (1983) blamed mainstream psychotherapy for the oppression of fat women and claimed that biology, not eating habits, is the main cause of fatness. This is an argument repeated by contemporary fat acceptance advocates (Robison and Carrier 2004). This argument rests on the well-documented empirical difficulties associated with trying to measure how much people actually eat. However, what this literature points to is the complexity of human body weight and the challenges that researchers face when trying to control for all the potentially relevant variables. Some studies support the idea that fat people eat more and some studies do not, but very few lead to firm conclusions either way about the general population. Claiming that over-eating plays little or no role in fatness is akin to arguing that a failure to show conclusively that motorcar emissions exacerbate global warming or increase asthma levels *proves* that emissions are benign. Motorcar emissions may or may not have these effects but an ambiguous set of research findings does not prove the case either way.

LETTING SCIENCE SPEAK

Although it is anything but an original insight, the point is worth reiterating: interested groups and individuals will seize on scraps of scientific evidence if they support their ideological position. They will do this even when the bulk of existing evidence does not support their view. This was the point I tried to make when asked in 2006 to contribute an article for a fat acceptance journal that, for reasons that will shortly become clear, I will not name. The intention of the journal had been to bring together articles by a number of the 'obesity sceptics' in a single edition. For my contribution, I decided to show how the words 'science' and 'truth' were used differently in the work of various sceptics. In short, I pointed out that while Jan Wright and I had argued in *The Obesity Epidemic* that obesity science had produced few reliable empirical truths, the more high-profile North American sceptics asserted that scientific truth was on their side. For example, Paul Campos (2004a), Glen Gaesser (2002) and others (e.g. Oliver 2006) constantly use words like 'myth', 'truth', 'lies' and 'liars' when writing about mainstream obesity science. *The Obesity Epidemic* argued that morality and ideology filled in the very large gaps created by a radically inconclusive scientific literature. For the North Americans, however, there were no gaps; objective scientific truth was there in the literature for any honest person who cared to look objectively at the 'evidence'. For example, around the time of the release of his book *The Obesity Myth*, Paul Campos published a series of articles in newspapers around the world under headlines like 'Big fat lie' and 'The big fat con story'. In one of these articles he wrote:

> What I have found may prove hard for some to swallow: save for exceptions involving truly extreme cases, the medical literature simply does not support the claim that higher than average weight is a significant independent health risk. What it actually demonstrates is, first, that the association between increased weight and increased health risk is weak, and disappears altogether when confounding variables are taken into account; and second, that public health programmes which attempt to make "overweight" and "obese" people thinner are, for a variety of reasons, likely to do more harm than good. In short, the current war on fat is an irrational outburst of cultural hysteria, unsupported by sound science.
>
> (Campos 2004b: 20)

That mainstream obesity science was suffering from 'cultural hysteria', as Campos puts it, is not an idea I support. Obesity scientists are not 'liars', involved in a 'con', and they are not, by and large, hysterical. How easy it is to dismiss those with whom we disagree by calling them bad and mad.

In developing this line of argument, my article was rejected on the grounds that the journal was not a forum for debate. It was explained to me that the journal was part of a movement whose mission was to promote a particular view of health and body weight. I want to be clear that I do not in any way begrudge a publication or its editor the right to make its own decisions for its own reasons. The editor of the journal has been a valuable public advocate for *The Obesity Epidemic* and is a thoughtful writer about obesity. Rather, I want simply to point out how assumed political and academic affinities (affinity seems to have been assumed by both parties in this instance) may turn out to be less straightforward. As I tried to show in the previous section, sometimes we may turn out to have greater affinity in unexpected quarters.

Another case in point relates to the work of the Oxford based Social Issues Research Centre (SIRC). In 2005 the centre produced *Obesity and the Facts: an analysis of data from the Health Survey for England 2003*. When I first became aware of the report in 2006 it seemed something of a godsend. Purporting to analyze published data from the UK's Department of Health, *Obesity and the Facts* argues that childhood body weights in the UK changed very little between the years 1993 and 2003. It claims that UK health authorities have erred by using outdated childhood weight distribution curves based only on UK data and which fail to take into account the upward secular trend in children's height. If, instead, more recently published distribution curves based on international data are used, the report argues that the idea of a childhood obesity crisis begins to look fanciful. For example, it claims that:

> The average weight of boys aged 3–15 years in 1995 was 32.0kg. In 2003 it was 31.9kg. For girls the figures were 32.0kg and 32.4 kg respectively.
> The average 15 year old boy weighed 60.7kg in 2003, compared with 58.8kg in 1995. For 15 year old girls the figures were 58.9kg and 58.5kg respectively.
>
> (SIRC 2005: 2)

The authors write:

> We can conclude from these figures that there have been no significant changes in the average weights of children over nearly a decade. This can be taken as evidence that there has been no "epidemic" of weight gain, since an epidemic would certainly have affected average weights.
>
> (SIRC 2005: 3)

And later:

> With these data before us, it is hard to understand why so much of the emphasis and related investment in public policy initiatives to tackle obesity has been directed towards children and young people—attacks

on consumption of "junk food", proposed restrictions on advertising of "sugary fatty foods"—when the problems are most evident in older generations.

(SIRC 2005: 9)

The potential usefulness of *Obesity and the Facts* for my own research and advocacy agendas seemed obvious. But I was also curious. Who or what is SIRC? The centre's web page says:

SIRC is an independent, not-for-profit organisation based in Oxford, UK. We conduct research on a wide range of social topics and combine robust qualitative and quantitative methods with innovative analysis and thinking.

(SIRC 2008b)

While this seems unremarkable enough, clicking 'About SIRC' reveals the following:

SIRC aims to provide a balanced, calm and thoughtful perspective on social issues, promoting open and rational debates based on evidence rather than ideology. In pursuit of this balanced perspective, SIRC conducts research on positive aspects of social behaviour as well as the more problematic aspects that are the focus of most social-science research.

(SIRC 2008a)

The alert reader will then notice that the first named member of SIRC's 'Panel of Advisors' is Desmond Morris, the well known zoologist whose most famous publication is perhaps *The Naked Ape* (1967). Morris was one of the founding figures of sociobiology, the scientific movement that emerged in the late 1960s and early 1970s and claimed to show that human behaviour, including gendered behaviour, was the result of Darwinian natural selection. Sociobiologists positioned their work as a critique of social constructionist and feminist social science because, they claimed, it showed that gendered behaviour was predominantly 'natural' rather than the product of culture or social relations. Morris' fellow members on the panel include anthropologists Robin Fox and Lionel Tiger whose 1980s and 1990s work articulated the extremes of biological determinism, famously lamenting that contraception wounded men's 'natural' position at the head of kinship groups by artificially liberating women from men's control. The centre's co-directors include Kate Fox, Robin Fox's daughter, a widely published social anthropologist, and Peter Marsh, an occasional co-author with Desmond Morris.

At this point, the meaning behind SIRC's claims to offer 'a balanced, calm and thoughtful perspective on social issues' and to conduct research 'on positive aspects of social behaviour as well as the more problematic aspects that are the focus of most social-science research' become clearer. Much of the research listed on SIRC's web pages takes a decidedly celebratory attitude to everyday life. For example, feminist scholars who have critiqued the dominance of male sports in Western culture will be interested in SIRC's commissioned report *The Impact of Sport on the Workplace* (SIRC 2006). The report's cover shows attractive young people in business dress, smiling and clapping as they (presumably) watch sport on an unseen screen. And contrary to commentators who have bemoaned the money, attention and cultural kudos given to elite sports people, *The Impact of Sport on the Workplace* recommends that employers create more opportunities for employees to watch, celebrate and talk about elite sport.

In short, the work of the SIRC represents a particular kind of critique of academic social science. Its members have led an assault on what they see as the undue influence of non-rational, evidence-free, ideological academic feminism and the carping of university based social scientists. Their view is that our social worlds are to a large extent given to us by our biological and cultural histories and that these should be judiciously respected, celebrated and preserved. As their self-description makes clear, they see themselves as a sober, scientific, objective voice in a culture preoccupied with risk and fear and inclined to believe the worst. SIRC's interest in obesity can be contextualized within this agenda. Their objection to obesity crisis rhetoric is that it pathologizes modern life and exaggerates the need for change.

From my perspective, members of the SIRC include authors of some of the most misguided and repugnant social science ever written. In particular, there could be few writers who have done more than Desmond Morris to popularize the idea that gender relations are biologically determined and that attempts, especially by feminists, to engineer change is both dangerous and futile.

Like my own work, SIRC's *Obesity and the Facts* has been largely ignored by mainstream medicine with only a small number of articles even bothering to dispute its findings. But, in the context of this chapter, this example raises an important question: what should our attitude to publications like *Obesity and the Facts* be? Most if not all of the contributors to this volume make either explicitly feminist or feminist influenced arguments about the 'obesity epidemic'. For many, their reasons for engaging in this debate rest in part on critiques of the alleged androcentric biases of mainstream science and medicine. These are critiques that members of SIRC are unlikely to have much sympathy for. But, like Furedi, they also draw heavily on analyses of obesity science written by other writers that, as far as I can see, they take on trust.

Of course, taking the findings of other researchers on trust is something that scholars in all fields do all of the time. We all cite research done by other people and we often have no choice but to trust they are telling the truth and that their conclusions are justified. No doubt there will be those who argue that this situation is easily remedied by scrutinising the data and methods of the works we cite. But this would be an impossibly time consuming business if we did it in all cases.

So my point here is that while many of us in the social sciences spend a lot of time thinking about the ideological biases of our enemies, there is no reason for us not to be equally vigilant about the ideological biases of our friends. Despite its apparent usefulness, I am inclined (perhaps unfairly) to suspect the efficacy of *Obesity and the Facts* because I know that much of the other work of its authors is ideologically compromised. I hasten to add that this does not mean that my suspicions are justified. Rather, what I think this highlights is the 'business-as-usual' acceptance of 'like-minded' friends' work, a practice which may actually be the life blood of all politically minded social science agendas, but particularly oppositional ones such as critical obesity studies. And while this is not a point likely ever to derail an academic project such as the one being prosecuted in this volume, it is, I think, a valuable counterpoint, as it were.

By way of a final example, I turn to the 2005-edited volume *Panic Nation: unpicking the myths we're told about food and health* (Feldman and Marks 2005). Edited by a prominent anaesthetist (Stanley Feldman) and clinical biochemist (Vincent Marks), *Panic Nation* consists of 30 mythbusting chapters across a wide range of medical and health controversies from salt, cholesterol, breast cancer screening to passive smoking. I heard Vincent Marks discussing the book on the radio around the time of its release. He was clearly a man of considerable age and spoke with the patrician tones we might stereotypically expect of a man who first studied medicine at Oxford in the late 1940s.

The volume itself opens with a portrait of Peraclesus (1493–1541), the 'father of modern toxicology' (Feldman and Marks 2005: ii), and proceeds in a similar and unfailingly self-serious tone to take the sword to what the editors see as the trendy and dim-witted health and medical myths of the modern age. The consistent line of the 30 chapters is that pressure groups and bad scientists have managed to grossly exaggerate the health risks of things like salt, sugar, cholesterol, fast food and passive smoking, as well as pseudo conditions like repetitive strain injury and stress-related illness. These same misguided groups have championed a wide range of useless, expensive and faddish pills, potions and interventions like food labelling, commercially available vitamins and minerals, complementary medicine, organic food and breast cancer screening. They are also responsible for scurrilously impugning the reputation of standard medical interventions like Hormone Replacement Therapy (HRT) and child immunization. By contrast, the chapters are exclusively pro-business; they give a clean bill of health to food additives, the use of pesticides and Genetically Modified (GM) food. Likewise, the air we breathe has never been cleaner and we really have nothing to worry about from mad cow disease.

Taken together, *Panic Nation* asks us to put our trust in two institutions: private enterprise and mainstream scientific (as opposed to fringe) medicine.

Our enemies are radical environmentalists, new-agists, vegetarians, feminists and health-and-fitness nuts, or what the editors collectively call 'pressure groups'. The tone of the book is exquisitely captured in Marks' chapter on 'healthy eating'. Here, the self-image of the book's authors as sage purveyors of scientific, time honoured truths, immune to the fashions and hysterias of the day, is all but spelt out.

> The famous food pyramid, introduced to simplify the healthy eating message and based upon 1980s dogma, is already outmoded and incorrect. What is the advice on healthy eating today? I believe that, as in the past, we should eat a variety of different foods from the dairy, grocer, baker, fruiterer, greengrocer and vintner, and somewhat less frequently from the fishmonger and butcher, in portion sizes and total quantity that ensures proper growth in children and the maintenance of a body mass index of around 20–25 in young adults and 23–27 in older adults. This coupled with moderate daily exercise, involves a lifestyle that becomes easier to practice once one understands the reason why it is good for one's health.
>
> (Marks 2005: 50–1)

It is difficult to know whether Marks' use of words like 'fruiterer', 'vintner' and 'fishmonger' is either quaintly and innocently anachronistic or assertively nostalgic and conservative. The message concerning the value of traditional wisdom ('as in the past') and moderation (as opposed to trendy fanaticism) in all things, though, is unmistakable.

Marks' chapter on obesity claims that the risks of obesity have been exaggerated, marshalling a similar set of arguments to the ones made by authors in this volume. But this is where similarities end. While the conference that led to this volume and the chapters themselves are almost entirely the work of female scholars, *Panic Nation*'s contributors are 18 men. More significantly, *Panic Nation* crafts its scepticism out of its allegiance to mainstream, 'respectable' medical science and its opposition to feminists and the enemies of big business. But in the present volume, feminist theory and politics as well as critiques of mainstream science provide the intellectual resources for questioning conventional wisdom about obesity. Same destination, diametrically opposed routes.

This is interesting because, as I mentioned above, there is a difference between sceptics like myself and Jan Wright and North American sceptics like Paul Campos and Glen Gaesser. Gard and Wright propose that even if we take mainstream science on its own terms, there are strong reasons to doubt the seriousness of the 'obesity epidemic'. In other words, mainstream science, even when conducted with the best of intentions, produces inconclusive results. For Campos and Gaesser, though, mainstream science is basically corrupt; it is only when we do 'good', 'unbiased' science that its true voice can be heard. And for Campos and Gasser the true voice of science tells us that mainstream science is lying about obesity. *Panic Nation*'s position is different again: mainstream obesity science is both trustworthy and the only way to produce robust and reliable truths. For these authors the enemies of truth come from outside science.

THE JOURNEY OR THE DESTINATION?

There are no signs that the 2007 defeat of the conservative government in Australia is likely to lead to a waning of the rhetorical 'war on obesity' in that country. Kevin Rudd's Labor party has promised to implement BMI tests for 4 year-old children when their parents present them for mandatory inoculations. In effect, in 2007, and without much fanfare, BMI testing became compulsory for Australian infants. In the media interviews I conducted about infant BMI testing, journalists fell into three camps. There were those who, like me, disliked the policy and worried about its impact on children. A second group saw it as common sense and were genuinely curious to know what objection I could possibly have. However, by far the majority seemed to come to the subject with an open mind, although I accept that this is probably the impression a well-trained journalist is supposed to give. My point here is that we should be careful not to accept Furedi's 'culture of fear' thesis uncritically. There is a tendency amongst those on the pessimistic liberal left *and* the libertarian right to bemoan the media's unquenchable thirst for bad news. In both camps the success of 'obesity epidemic' discourse is seen as symptomatic of a culture which runs on risk and fear and, therefore, *needs* crises and epidemics in order to function normally.

I think this is a mistaken view. My personal experience is that there is a great appetite for alternative viewpoints in the media and amongst people who have taken at least a passing interest in obesity as an issue. My purpose in this chapter has simply been to point out that populist and politically useful ideas are circulating in our culture. These ideas are waiting to be exploited. Sometimes these ideas are most closely associated with people we (regardless of who 'we' are) might normally have seen as natural enemies.

In short, I take it as a given that critical obesity scholars are interested in reducing the harm that uncontested talk of an obesity crisis will have in the world. My argument is that scholars are most effective when they are able to infiltrate and exploit a range of rhetorical and ideological traditions. However, as a scholar who came of age, so to speak, in the late 1990s and early 2000s, I noticed that rhetoric and ideology are often linked closely with academic identity; that is, young and older scholars alike were inclined to ask 'who are you? A Foucauldian? A poststructuralist? A positivist? A queer theorist?' In particular, my own academic disciplines— education and physical education—have relied on caricatures of more conservative intellectual traditions. This means that because many scholars do not understand conservative arguments they are not able to use them, let alone critique them. In their hearts, they probably know that the world is not much interested in whether 'obesity discourse' contributes to the 'medicalization' of society or 'marginalizes' particular 'subjectivities', but they are unsure what else to say. I have lost count of the number of times I have heard scholars talk about the 'medicalization' of society as if their listeners would automatically recognize this as a bad thing. In other words, one of the most important mistakes scholars must avoid is to load (that is, reify) their conceptual landscape with political and moral import.

The answer to this is trying to understand how other intellectual traditions operate and using them strategically; in effect, speaking other languages other than one's own. In part this means confronting the emptiness of calling oneself a poststructuralist or a Foucauldian or any other academic label that calls upon us to think and act 'consistently' because we think we are who we say we are. Taking up the theme of this volume more explicitly, I think this also means that we need to be careful about freezing the term 'biopedagogy' such that it becomes a pejorative code word with which to brand any discussion about obesity that does not conform to the party line. After all, a logical conclusion of the arguments I have presented here is that critical obesity researchers should understand and be able to employ the techniques of biopedagogy for their own subversive ends.

We might also remember that a 'culture of fear' is one where intellectual consistency counts for little. Ulrich Beck was right about risk being an acid that dissolves old political alliances because, like desire, being in a state of fear bypasses our stated political and intellectual affiliations. Obesity is an utterly plastic social issue and one's orientation to it is much more a matter of visceral belief than cerebral truth, a point that should help to prepare us for the promiscuous intellectual advocacy this issue calls for.

REFERENCES

Beck, U. (1992) *Risk Society*, Sage: London.

Burkeman, O. (2006) 'Food fight', *The Guardian*, 22 April: 31.

Campos, P. (2004a) *The Obesity Myth: Why America's Obsession with Weight is Hazardous to Your Health*, New York: Gotham Books.

Campos, P. (2004b) 'Why our fears about fat are misplaced', *New Scientist*, 182(2445): 20.

Campos, P.A., Saguy, P., Ernsberger, E., Oliver and Gaesser, G. (2006) 'The epidemiology of overweight and obesity: public health crisis or moral panic', *International Journal of Epidemiology*, 35(1): 55–60.

CBS News (2006) 'Obesity an "international scourge"', 3 September: retrieved 26 June 2007, from http://www.cbsnews.com/stories/2006/09/03/health/main1962961.shtml

Critser, G. (2000) 'Let them eat fat', *Harper's Magazine*, March: 41–7.

Critser, G. (2003) *Fat Land: How Americans Became the Fattest People in the World*, London: Penguin Books.

Feldman, S. and Marks, V. (eds) (2005) *Panic Nation: Unpicking the Myths We're Told About Food and Health*, London: John Blake.

Fumento, M. (1997) *The Fat of the Land: The Obesity Epidemic and How Overweight Americans Can Help Themselves*, New York: Viking.

Furedi, F. (1997) *Culture of Fear: Risk Taking and the Morality of Low Expectation*, London: Cassell.

Gaesser, G.A. (2002) *Big Fat Lies: The Truth About your Weight and Your Health*, Carlsbad: Gurze Books.

Gard, M. and Wright, J. (2005) *The Obesity Epidemic*, London: Routledge.

jonjayray (2005) 'Fat and Fiction', weblog post, *Political Correctness Watch*, 13 June: retrieved 11 March 2008, from http://pcwatch.blogspot.com/2005_06_01_archive.html

Marks, V. (2005) 'Healthy Eating', in S. Feldman and V. Marks (eds) *Panic Nation: Unpicking the Myths We're Told About Food and Health*, London: John Blake.

Mayer, V.F. (1983) 'The Fat Illusion', in L. Schoenfielder and B. Wieser (eds) *Shadow on a Tightrope: Writings by Women on Fat Oppression*, San Francisco: Spinsters/Aunt Lute.

Oliver, J.E. (2006) *Fat Politics: The Real Story Behind America's Obesity Epidemic*, Oxford: Oxford University Press.

Political Correctness Watch (2005) *Political Correctness Watch: the creeping dictatorship of the left*. Weblog: retrieved 11 March 2008, from http://pcwatch.blogspot.com

Robison, J. and Carrier, K. (2004) *The Spirit and Science of Holistic Health*, Bloomington: AuthorHouse.

Schlosser, E. (2001) *Fast Food Nation: What the All-American Meal is Doing to the World*, London: Allen Lane.

SIRC (2005) *Obesity and the Facts: An Analysis of Data from the Health Survey for England 2003*, retrieved 10 July 2008, from http://www.sirc.org/obesity/obesity_and_the_facts.shtml

SIRC (2006) *The Impact of Sport on the Workplace*, retrieved 10 July 2008, from http://www.sirc.org/publik/sport_and_the_workplace.shtml

SIRC (2008a) 'About SIRC', retrieved 10 July 2008, from http://www.sirc.org/about/about.html

SIRC (2008b) 'Welcome to the Social Issues Research Centre', retrieved 10 July 2008, from http://www.sirc.org/index.html

4 Bio-Citizenship
Virtue Discourses and the Birth of the Bio-Citizen

Christine Halse

IN THE BEGINNING . . .

This chapter describes the emergence of a new species of human being—the bio-citizen. The bio-citizen is a product of an era of escalating anxiety in the public imagination about an international pandemic of overweight and obesity. A Google of the word 'obesity' generates millions of references that increase in number on a daily basis e.g., 32,600,000 items (3 January 2008), 33,600,000 (9 June 2008). No-one, media commentators warn, has been left unscathed by the 'obesity epidemic':

> [m]ake no mistake: the dreaded obesity epidemic that is everywhere in the news is not restricted to any race, creed, ethnicity or slice of the socioeconomic supersized pie. As recent studies reveal, virtually every group known to democracy is getting fatter.
>
> (Angier 2000: 1)

Medical experts have described the twenty-first century as an 'obesogenic environment' (Prioietto and Baur 2004), and the moral panic about an 'obesity epidemic' has been taken up by the disciplines, governments, and their surrogates (Campos, Saguy, Ernsberger, Oliver, and Gaesser 2006). It is evident in the funding priorities of medical and scientific research; the reform agendas of social agents such as health services, education and the media; in the programs and policies of governments and national bodies such as the United States of America (USA) Center for Disease Control (CDC) and in the surveillance activities of supranational agencies such as the World Health Organisation (WHO).

The rhetoric of an 'obesity epidemic' has spawned a global weight-loss industry that provides diet products, programs, counsellors and advisors to help people secure the ideal of a normative body weight. Local and online diet clubs have constructed new communities whose members are joined by the shared desire to lose weight. New diet regimes and scrutiny of the weight of movie and music glitterati are the staple of popular and women's magazines, and internationally syndicated reality TV programs like *The Biggest Loser* have turned weight loss into a competitive, public sport.

Few cultural practices or organizations have escaped the growing obsession with overweight and obesity. Fast food outlets like McDonalds have succumbed and now provide customers with low-calorie foods options: no-fat muffins, 'McLean' burgers, low-fat milkshakes, salads and fruit. Even the World Pie Eating Championship has abandoned its tradition of eating as many meat and potato pies as possible in 3 minutes. Now competitors eat one regulation 12 cm pie as quickly as possible—and a vegetarian option is provided. According to organizers, the move was in response to 'government inspired guidelines on obesity' (No Author 2006c).

Scholars have challenged the plausibility of the obesity epidemic and accused the media, medical and scientific experts, and public health officials of exaggerating the negative effects of overweight and obesity on health (Campos 2004; Gard and Wright 2005; Oliver 2005). The controversy surrounding the 'obesity epidemic' has also become politicized. Illustrative are the campaigns by conservative organizations such as the Centre for Consumer Freedom (CCF), a non-profit, US coalition of restaurants, food companies and consumers whose goal is to oppose:

> [t]he growing cabal of "food cops", health care enforcers, militant activists, meddling bureaucrats, and violent radicals who think they know "what's best for you" [and] are pushing against our basic freedoms.
>
> (The Centre for Consumer Freedom 2008)

With this end in sight, the CCF has lobbied against legislation that seeks to control the eating and weight of the country's population, in the name of protecting personal responsibility, individual autonomy and consumer choice.

UNRAVELLING THE BODY (MASS INDEX)

What has made the idea of an obesity epidemic *possible* is the development of a discourse of a normative Body Mass Index (BMI) as the '"virtuous mean" to which we should *all* aspire' (Burry 1999: 610). BMI is the mathematical (re)presentation of weight that is calculated by dividing a person's weight by the square of his or her height. Belgian statistician, Adolphe Quetelet, developed the formula for BMI in the 1800s and the idea of a prudential, BMI norm has progressively colonized the policies, practices and procedures for measuring and documenting weight. The US military first used BMI tables during the Civil War and later to exclude underweight recruits from the Korean War. In the 1980s, the World Health Organization set international definitions for BMI: underweight (less than BMI 20); average (BMI 20–24.9); overweight (BMI 25–29.9); and obese (BMI 30+). In 1998, the National Institutes of Health in the USA aligned their weight definitions with the WHO guidelines, lowering the normal/ overweight BMI cut-off in the USA from BMI 27.8 to BMI 25. BMI is now the standard benchmark used by clinical and public health offices, medical organizations, researchers and policy makers to calculate, describe and compare the weight of individuals and populations.

At least in part, the persuasive capacity and take-up of the discourse of a normative BMI lies in its simplicity and its rhetoric of scientism. BMI deploys the language of scientific positivism to invoke an aura of truth, trustworthiness and transparency, and is easily calculated without the help of specialist tools. These tactics represent BMI as an objective fact that is devoid of personal prejudice or subjective value, and locate the discourse of BMI in the 'science' of the body.

But BMI is a slippery, contested creature. It is premised on the assumption that there is an identifiable 'normal' weight that is 'true' across genders and across different cultural, socio-economic and geographical groups. Yet even scientific experts who advocate the use of BMI as an epidemiological tool concede that it is an 'arbitrary' measure (James, Leach, Kalamara, and Shayeghi 2001: 228). BMI describes the relationship between net weight and height but it fails to take into account differences in physical frame or proportions of fat, muscle and bone mass, cartilage or fluid retention. It was this imprecision that triggered controversy when the World Health Organization (WHO) decreed the normative BMI to be between 20 and 24.9. There was an immediate outcry in Asian countries, with a call for 'a more limited range for normal BMIs (i.e. 18.5 to 22.9 kg/m² rather than 18.5 to 24.9 kg/m²)' because Asian populations have smaller frames and greater health risks at a lower weight than people of non-Asian backgrounds (James et al. 2001: 228).

Nor is the relationship between BMI and ill health straightforward. Genetics and activity levels are important mediating factors for good health, and British researchers warn that a normative BMI can disguise the *nature* of weight because many slim people can store dangerous levels of fat in their bodies that can trigger heart conditions and diabetes: '[p]eople shouldn't be happy just because they look thin . . . you can have a lot of fat internally, which can have a detrimental effect on your health' (No Author 2006d: 3).

UNRAVELLING THE VIRTUE DISCOURSE OF A NORMATIVE BMI

Nevertheless, the notion of a normative BMI has survived as a 'virtue discourse' that describes and defines weight, bodies and individuals. Virtue discourses are sets of values, beliefs, practices and behaviours that establish regimes of truth and shape subjects and subjectivities by articulating and constructing particular behaviours and qualities as worthy, desirable and necessary virtues.

What distinguishes the work of 'virtue discourses' from other discourses is that they 'configure virtue as an open-ended condition: a state of excellence that has no boundaries or exclusions' (Halse, Honey and Boughtwood 2007: 220). This infinite open-endedness means that it is not possible to be *too* industrious or *too* diligent about taking up the dietary practices, exercise regimes, pharmaceutical and cosmetic interventions necessary to manage one's weight and maintain a 'normal' BMI.

The virtue discourse of a normative BMI is also highly moralistic because it invokes and relies on binaries that ascribe 'opposing moral attributes to each side of the binary that seem natural, logical and fair' (Halse 2006: 107). Thus, in societies where slenderness is idealized and desired, a low BMI is aligned with self-discipline and restraint and a high BMI (overweight or obesity) is the binary 'Other'—the physical manifestation of self-indulgence and a lack of self-discipline and moral fortitude. Such binary constructions move beyond a discourse of healthism in which slenderness is equated with fitness and health by constituting slenderness as a *necessary state of being* to avoid fatness—a socially repugnant state that is a 'metonym for laziness and ugliness' (Halse et al. 2007: 228) and an indicator of some troubling physical or psychological pathology warranting oversight, disciplining and correction.

The virtue discourse of a normative BMI is communicated through the images and messages of popular culture, advertising and the media; films and television programs; and the authoritative messages circulated by the weight-loss industry, health education, school curricula, and the medical profession. It permeates the pores of individuals and populations by immersion in and habituation to its terms and moral values, and through political tactics that define desirable and approved behaviour. Individuals who take up the discourse by keeping (virtuously) slender are congratulated and rewarded. They are recognized and applauded by family, friends, and colleagues; venerated by advertisers and in the popular press; and commended in the commentaries of health and medical authorities. Those who are non-compliant and overweight or obese are likely to suffer social exclusion and alienation. They are more likely to face higher health care and insurance charges, to have physical difficulty traveling in airplanes or public transport where space is confined, and to be excluded from areas of state employment. In the United Kingdom and most Australian, New Zealand and US states, compliance with designated BMI cut-offs is a criterion for admission to the armed forces, Fire Brigade, Special Constabulary, and Port Authority Police. Maintaining the required BMI cut-off is also a condition for *continued* employment in the army, police and fire brigades, and government sponsored health and weight loss programs have been introduced in some countries, including New Zealand, Turkey and Thailand, to help the police and firefighters get into shape (Anon. 2005a 2005b; Devechi, Gülbayrak, Oğuzöncül, and Açik 2004).

Researchers, media commentators and medical experts also warn that overweight or obese individuals are statistically more likely to experience lower living standards, lower levels of social, economic, political and educational understanding, and a higher incidence of social disadvantage (Burry 1999). As British research published in the *Sydney Morning Herald* pronounced: '[t]he fatter you were, the less you earned, with lower-paid clerical workers nine times more likely to be overweight (75 per cent) than those at upper management level (8 per cent)' (Delaney 2007).

Through the operation of bio-power—the regulation of subjects by the state—the virtue discourse of a normative BMI constructs subjects who have a material investment in maintaining the discourse's terms. For instance, the police in Queensland, Australia, have argued for the reintroduction of height and weight restrictions for police to improve the physical presence of beat police because 'physically challenged' police put 'themselves and their colleagues at greater risk of assault' (Ironside 2008). Similarly, in the USA, a succession of legal cases has upheld the right of government agencies to dismiss overweight or obese firefighters, police and other employees (Perritt 2002; Roehling 1999).

While not all individuals are subjugated at the same time or in the same way, the pervasiveness of the virtue discourse of a normative BMI shapes citizens' self-understandings and self-techniques so that it is taken up as 'a mode of personal self-regulation [and] internal constraint on the conduct of the self' (Halse et al. 2007: 223). In this way, the virtue discourse of a normative BMI incorporates the 'outside' world (values and beliefs) into the 'inside' (psyche and bodily practices) of individuals. Deleuze (2000: 118–9) captures the fusion of the 'inside' and 'outside' in his notion of the human subject as the outside folded in—an immanently social, political and embedded subject:

> [t]he outside is not a fixed limit but a moving matter animated by peristaltic movements, folds and foldings that together make up an inside: they are not something other than the outside, but precisely the inside of the outside.

However, the political effects of the virtue discourse of a normative BMI do moral mischief. By differentiating between those who are and are not acceptable and approved sorts of human beings within its own moral schema, the virtue discourse of a normative BMI works to 'establish what qualifies as "being"' (Bulter 1993: 188): thin/fat, normal/abnormal, virtuous/sinful, worthy/unworthy.

The discourse also has a more sinister effect. By deploying a mechanical, statistical procedure to calculate BMI, individuals and groups are reduced to numeric entities that become amenable to categorization and comparison. Deleuze (1992: 4) has described the effects of administratively numerating bodies: '[it] individualizes and masses together [and] constitutes those over whom it exercises power into a body and molds the individuality of each member of that body'. Through mathematical reduction, the assignment/adoption of BMI metaphorically erases the heart, soul and history of human subjects, substituting in its place a (numeric) entity devoid of personal or social identity on which the state and its allies can inscribe a new persona—that of the (virtuous) bio-citizen.

CITIZENSHIP AND THE BIO-CITIZEN

The bio-citizen has emerged as a new sociological and biological benchmark for describing, categorising and differentiating between human beings and human societies. This new species of human being—the bio-citizen— extends Rose and Novas' (Rose and Novas 2003) theory of biological citizenship by which somatic individuality—physical ailments, illnesses and genetics—fashions relations between individuals and shapes their engagement in different political, electronic and social communities. The bio-citizen is a more complex persona because s/he has come into being by welding the body onto the social, cultural, economic and political responsibilities of citizenship and the state.

The bio-citizen is grounded in a concept of citizenship that moves beyond simplistic definitions of citizenship as a legal status and 'bundle of entitlements and obligations which constitute individuals as fully fledged members of a socio-political community' (Turner 1994: 1). Rather, the bio-citizen resurrects a notion of citizenship that had its origin in the Athenian politics of Ancient Greece. This was a time when citizenship centred on the polis, an individual's private life was considered a public matter, and the obligations of the individual were inextricably bound to the daily operation and organisation of the community. Citizenship was not merely a matter of individual rights granted by virtue of political membership to a community. Rather, citizenship was based on a set of relations between the individual and the state that involved a conscious contribution by the citizenry to improving the life and well-being of the community by actively demonstrating the moral virtues of the citizen—wisdom, temperance, justice and courage. The 'good' citizen is therefore an 'active' citizen, and active citizenship is the means by which one both commits to and becomes immersed in and part of the social world of a community.

Nikolas Rose (1989/1999) argues that this political rationality was revived during the first half of the twentieth century when the citizen was transformed from a subject with legal and constitutional rights and duties into a social being whose existence was articulated in the language of social responsibilities and collective solidarity.

> The individual was to be integrated into society in the form of the citizen with social needs in a contract in which individual and society would have mutual claims and obligations. Each individual was to become an active agent in the maintenance of health and efficient

polity, exercising a reflexive scrutiny of personal, domestic, and familial conduct. (Rose 1999: 228)

While active citizenship is central to the identity of the new bio-citizen, her/his identity also derives from the disembodied, rational subject of liberal humanism, a universal ethic of justice and a notion of the common good. These ideas had their roots in the writings of Plato, Aristotle, and Cicero but their contemporary meanings were developed by philosopher John Rawls (1971/1999) who argued that the common good involves an implicit social contract (agreement) between individuals and the state that equal access to certain general social conditions advantages all members of a society. This social contract was necessary to serve the common good and construct a well-ordered society in an increasingly complex, interdependent world (Andre and Velasquez 1992). In this schema, what *counts* as virtuous, moral actions are those that serve the interests of the individual *and* all others in any society. Thus, for the bio-citizen, failure to control one's weight makes one a 'bad' citizen by ignoring the interests of the common good needed for a well-ordered society.

THE BIO-CITIZEN, THE COMMON GOOD
AND THE WELL-ORDERED SOCIETY

The first obligation of the bio-citizen to the common good is to take personal responsibility for the physical care of oneself. Maintaining one's weight within the BMI 'norm' is crucial to meeting this goal. Burry (1999: 610), for example, enunciates this philosophy when he instructs, in the *Journal of the Australian Medical Association*: '[c]ontrol of weight, no matter that some have a genetically determined potential to acquire and retain more weight in comparison with others, remains a matter of self-control and personal responsibility'.

Media and consumer groups have latched onto the messy matter of weight as a personal responsibility. In Australia, for instance, *The Age* newspaper has decreed: '[a] healthy diet and exercise regime is an individual responsibility' (No Author 2006b). In the United States, the Journal of the Diabetes Association of America, reporting on the flurry of unsuccessful litigation against fast food companies for producing flavoursome food without adequate health warnings of the dangers of consumption, cited medical experts who cautioned: 'personal responsibility is still the key to diet and exercise and other positive health activities' (No Author 2006a). At an international level, key questions examined by the 18th International Congress of Nutrition in Durban in 2005 included: Is the global obesity pandemic the responsibility of the individual or governments? Who is to blame? Who should be responsible for reversing the trend?

Reconfiguring personal responsibility as a social responsibility ratchets up the burden on and accountability of the individual for the well-being of society, but becoming a (virtuous) bio-citizen involves *more* than taking responsibility for ensuring that one's weight stays within the BMI 'norm'. It is a responsibility to care for oneself *in order to* care for one's offspring and family—including any unborn children. For example, scientists warn that overweight mothers put their unborn children at risk because maternal obesity transmits the 'obesity gene' to offspring and is linked to miscarriage, preterm birth, stillbirth and neo-natal deaths (BBC 2008). Similarly, anti-obesity campaigners argue that ensuring 'we can get women at the right weight at pre-conception' means that 'we can prevent this whole obesity issue' (Hagan 2008). Aspiring mothers are also urged to stay slender *to defend* their children against the *future possibility* of being overweight because 'obesity is more likely in offspring if parents are obese' (Burry 1999: 609).

The moral imperative to care for one's weight *in order to care for others* does not abate after the birth of children. Medical experts and the media urge parents 'to shape up' by eating healthy foods, exercising and watching their weight because they are 'role models' for their children (Hagan 2008; McDowell 2008). Parents are advised to set 'a good example by sitting down to breakfast' because 'the more often an adolescent [has] breakfast, the lower the BMI' (Bakalar 2008). Parents can draw on a bevy of paediatric dieticians, medical specialists, advisers and counsellors for support in helping their children lose weight. Or they can go online where sites such as 'My Overweight Child' offer 'tips, strategies and guidance for parents of overweight kids' (No Author 2008a). If these strategies fail, the Surgeon General of the United States recommends a 'family-centric weight management program' with nutrition lessons, exercise sessions and mandatory parental involvement (Hunter 2008). Similarly, the medical profession—including the esteemed Mayo Clinic urges parents to '[m]ake weight loss a family affair' to beat childhood obesity (Mayo Foundation for Medical Education and Research 2006; Prioietto and Baur 2004). As a last resort, parents can secure their children's future by sending them to 'weight-loss boarding school' so that they learn 'to eat right, exercise more and fight the genetics that have placed them among the millions of children who struggle with obesity' (Bompey and Wilson 2008).

Recalcitrant parents who fail to control their own weight and that of their children leave themselves open to being ridiculed, blamed and decried as 'bad parents'. Or they are punished by the state with the loss of child custody and parental rights, as in the case of 3 year-old Anamarie Martinez-Regino. Weighing in at 54 kilograms, the 3 ft 6 ins tall Anamarie was three times heavier than an average 3 year-old; and she was removed from her parent's custody by the government of New Mexico, USA, 'because they could not control her weight' (No Author 2002).

The responsibility of the bio-citizen involves more than a social contract to care for one's own weight and the weight of one's family. It is a responsibility to care for the health and economic well-being of others in the community and the nation. The idea that overweight and obesity causes economic damage is so widespread that it has become conventional wisdom (Gard and Wright 2005). Medical authorities and the media warn that failing to care for one's weight by becoming overweight or obese can cause a litany of potentially avoidable health problems, including sleep disorders, high blood pressure, diabetes, heart disease, stroke, arthritis, cancer, and poor reproductive health. These undermine the 'healthy functioning of the general community' (Burry 1999: 610) and place an unwarranted strain on a nation's health-care system (No Author 2006b). The overweight and obese also require expensive, super-sized equipment that place additional burdens on the finances of governments and health agencies. For example, the State government of New South Wales, in Australia, recently:

> had to buy three additional super-sized ambulances, at $150,000 each, in order to cope with those people who are so fat they cannot fit inside a standard ambulance. They are designed for people who weigh at least 180 kilograms. Moving these patients can take up to 5 hours, and require the assistance of the police, fire-fighters, and SES volunteers . . . and hospitals are being forced to purchase special hydraulic lifting equipment to transfer obese people onto hospital beds. Extra large medical examination machines are needed, such as Computerized Tomograph (CT) and Magnetic Resonance Imagers (MRI), as the obese do not fit into the standard ones.
>
> (Smith 2008)

Because of the crisis caused by an overburdened health care system, ethicists have urged society to replace the current '"ethic of individual rights" with an "ethic of the common good"' (Andre and Velasquez 1992). But failing to care for one's weight is also blamed for causing nations other, unnecessary financial burdens. The Australian government has placed the financial cost of obesity in the region of $3.7 billion per year (Obesity Commission 2008) but a study commissioned by Diabetes Australia estimated the cost of increased expenditure on health *plus* the loss of economic productivity due to weight-related ill-health costs the community approximately $20.7 billion per annum (Uhlmann 2006).

It is also contended that failing to care for one's weight represents a threat to national security. According to a study by the US National Academy of Sciences and the Subcommittee on Military Weight Management, the increase in obesity in the USA:

> decreases the pool of individuals eligible for recruitment into military services, and it decreases the retention of new recruits. Almost 80 per cent of recruits who exceed the military accession weight-for-height standards at entry leave the military before they complete their first

term of enlistment. This in turn increases the cost of recruitment and training. These issues threaten the long-term welfare and readiness of the US.

(Subcommittee on Military Weight Management and
Committee on Military Nutrition Research 2004: 1)

Through such political strategies, the virtue discourse of a normative BMI constructs a moral universe in which *being* and *being recognisable* as a virtuous (bio) citizen requires active, demonstrable care for one's own weight and the weight of particular and generalized 'Others' in society (see Benhabib 1987). As Samantha Murray discusses in this book, controlling one's weight is constituted as the ethical responsibility to society of a virtuous (bio) citizen.

Thus, in contrast to the lazy, inert, self-absorbed subject—the 'bad' citizen implicated in the social and political rhetoric of an obesity epidemic—the model bio-citizen is a public-minded, socially responsible individual who is concerned about the common good and well-being of society. S/he adheres to the social contract between the individual and state by renouncing irresponsible weight-related behaviours as an active demonstration of care for the health and economic well-being of self, family and nation.

THE BIO-CITIZEN AND THE NATION STATE

The emergence of the bio-citizen (re)configures the relationship between individuals and collective social groupings. While the rhetoric of the obesity epidemic may not 'differentiate between particular social groups' (Gard and Wright 2005: 19), the *effects,* practices and technologies entangled in the virtue discourse of a normative BMI *do* differentiate and deliberately and actively *seek* to do so by elevating BMI to a descriptor and definer of human difference across social, cultural, political, economic and geographic axes.

This phenomenon is explicit in the obesity league tables that are gathered and circulated by government bodies, health authorities and social agencies, and periodically reproduced by the popular press. Across the globe, obesity league tables serve as a proxy for the health and economic well-being of local, national and international populations. At the local level, for example, in Australia's most densely populated state, New South Wales (NSW), media reports of the *Tenth Annual Health Report* told of the increased risk of premature death 'due to potentially avoidable causes' of overweight and obesity, and were accompanied by maps that highlighted the geographic and socio-economic regions where the average BMI was above the norm.

At a national level, the third annual report of 'The Trust for America's Health', entitled *F as in Fat: How Obesity Policies are Failing America*

(Trust for America's Health 2007) ranked obesity by state using data from the Centre for Disease Control and Prevention. Colorado had the country's lowest rate of obesity (16.9 per cent) but the survey identified the most economically disadvantaged, poorest areas in the South as home to nine of the country's 10 most obese states, with Mississippi (29.5 per cent) in first place followed by Alabama and West Virginia (Trust for America's Health 2007).

At the supranational level, the Noncommunicable Disease Surveillance (NCD) program conducted by the WHO collects national information about weight and develops country-based, comparative profiles as part of a global surveillance strategy to track country-level trends. How countries fare in the international weight stakes inevitably triggers national and international publicity and scrutiny, with journals like *Forbes Magazine* eager to profile the 'World's Fattest Countries' and to distribute national shame (Streib 2007).

While statistical surveillance of the population's weight through obesity league tables *appears* innocent—monitoring the weight of populations to improve the health of individuals and communities—they function as a sort of modern-day panopticon. Medical authorities, for example, have applauded the use of BMI to standardize classification of those who are overweight and obese because it enables 'comparable analysis of prevalence rates worldwide' and the gathering of 'comparative data from different countries, to depict secular changes in the epidemic, and, as noted, to help prepare a scheme for clinical management' (James et al. 2001: 228–9). Moreover, the technology of national and international weight surveillance has spawned a new transnational class of organizations that are devoted to sustaining the disciplinary regimes of the virtue discourse of a normative BMI. These include: the International Association for the Study of Obesity (IASO) and its policy arm, the International Obesity Task Force; the Global Prevention Alliance; and HOPE (Health Promotion through Obesity Prevention in Europe).

Far from dissolving social, cultural and economic differences, obesity league tables reshape how geographical spaces are conceptualized, defined and described, thereby reconfiguring understandings of local, national and international difference. Asserting a 'truth discourse', that a BMI outside the statistical 'norm' constitutes a social, economic and/or health problem, legitimates the intervention, disciplining and control of individuals and populations by states and their surrogates. Direct intervention and control by the state—as in the case of Anamarie Martinez-Regino—is evident in a number of domains and is symptomatic of what Deleuze (1992) described as the progression from disciplinary societies to societies of control. In the USA, for example, at least eight states have banned trans fats from schools (No Author 2008c); North Carolina, Florida, and other states have legislated to make physical education mandatory for all elementary school students (No Author 2007a 2008b); and federal legislators in the House of Representatives have advocated including physical education in the *No Child Left Behind (NCLB) Act (2001)*:

> The bill would add physical education to the multiple measures for determining accountability under NCLB, offering schools another way to meet their adequate yearly progress while promoting physical activity and nutritional education for students. States would be measured on their progress toward meeting a national goal for required physical education recommended by the Centers for Disease Control of 150 minutes per week in elementary schools and 225 minutes per week for students in middle and high schools. School districts and states would also be asked to report on students' physical activity and help promote healthy lifestyles.
>
> (No Author 2007b)

In short, obesity league tables function as a bio-political line of force in the armoury of bio-power—a regime of knowledge and authority over the physicality of individual and collective human vitality that is considered 'desirable, legitimate and efficacious' (Rabinow and Rose 2003: 2) by the governments and supranational agencies. The irony is that obesity league tables deploy a homogenising logic of sameness—the virtue discourse of a normative BMI—yet they work to make collective differences visible and distinct by grafting BMI onto the geographic and socio-economic profile of nations in ways that define and differentiate between populations by aligning weight with the social, racial, cultural and/or economic profile of a nation-state.

THE BIO-CITIZEN AND THE FUTURE . . .

As a result, citizenship is no longer coterminous with nationality but with the bodily practices of communities within the geographic boundary of the nation-state. Conflating responsibility for BMI with national geography positions the bio-citizen in the corporeal practices of identity. It grafts the body onto politics by physically differentiating between citizens along local, national and international geographical and political planes. The United Nations' *Declaration on the Elimination of All Forms of Racial Discrimination (1963)* banned discrimination by race, class or gender, and this principle has been enshrined through government legislation and laws in the majority of liberal, democratic societies. In contrast, the emergence of the bio-citizen represents a conceptual continuation of the eugenics movement of the eighteenth and nineteenth centuries that defined and differentiated between individuals and groups according to their physical characteristics, race, phrenology and/or genetic lineage.

Because governments and their agents have committed intense political energy and considerable financial resources to constructing the bio-citizen, the virtue discourse of a normative BMI is not an innocent bystander in choreographing the future. But what has been buried in the jetsam and flotsam of its wake are bigger, more difficult issues: hunger; poverty; physical abuse; lack of fresh water, medical care and education; discrimination and inequalities; social and economic disadvantage. A cynic might wonder if this is a stratagem—a bio-political ruse—by governments and their agents to deflect the citizenry's attention from the social justice issues that continue to blight the lives of individuals and the well-being of communities and nations. Whether this state of affairs is by design or circumstance, what remains unclear are the sorts of political strategies that will effectively subvert the virtue discourse of a normative BMI, rectify its effects and fracture the logic and identity of the bio-citizen.

However, even the act of *thinking* and *naming* the bio-citizen is a transgressive and potentially transformative act. As Deleuze reminds us, thinking involves the violent confrontation with reality that makes it possible to rupture the control of reality, to alter what we think is possible, and to become different sorts of human beings and citizens (Deleuze 1992).

REFERENCES

Andre, C. and Velasquez, M. (1992) 'The common good', *Issues in Ethics*, 5(1): retrieved 8 June 2008, from http://www.scu.edu/ethics/publications/iie/v5n1/common.html

Angier, N. (2000) 'Who is fat? It depends on culture', *The New York Times*, 7 November: retrieved 7 November 2000, from http://query.nytimes.com/gst/fullpage.html?res=980CE2DE1339F934A35752C1A9669C8B63

Anon. (2005a) *Fat Thai Police Ordered to Reduce Weight*, retrieved 1 June 2008, from http://www.salon.com/news/2005/06/21/thai/

Anon. (2005b) 'Health watch', *Police News*, 38(4): 81: retrieved 1 June 2008 from http://www.policeassn.org.nz/communications/newspdf/May05.pdf

Bakalar, N. (2008) 'Mom was right indeed!', *New York Times, Deccan Herald*, 29 April. Retrieved 12 May 2008, from http://www.deccanherald.com/Content/Apr222008/snt2008042163930.asp

BBC (2008) 'Stillbirth rate not coming down', retrieved 12 May 2008, from http://news.bbc.co.uk/2/hi/health/7388285.stm

Benhabib, S. (1987) 'The Generalised Other and the Concrete Other: The Kohlberg-Gilliam Controversy and Feminist Theory', in S. Benhabib and D. Cornell (eds) *Feminism as Critique: On the Politics of Gender*, Minneapolis: University of Minnesota Press.

Bompey, N. and Wilson, A. (2008) 'North Carolina school on front lines of childhood obesity fight', *Wausau Daily Herald*, 5 May: retrieved 12 May 2008, from http://www.wausaudailyherald.com/apps/pbcs.dll/article?AID=/20080505/WDH04/805050332/1619

Bulter, J. (1993) *Bodies that Matter: On the Discursive Limits of Sex*, New York: Routledge.

Burry, J. (1999) 'Obesity and virtue. Is staying lean a matter of ethics? Self-control of one's own weight might be described as a form of bioethics', *Medical Journal of Australia*, 171: 609–10.

Campos, P. (2004) *The Obesity Myth*, New York: Gotham Books.

Campos, P., Saguy, A., Ernsberger, P., Oliver, E. and Gaesser, G. (2006) 'The epidemiology of overweight and obesity: public health crisis or moral panic? Point—Counterpoint', *International Journal of Epidemiology*, 35(1): 55–60.

Delaney, B. (2007) 'Fat end the wedge between classes', *Sydney Morning Herald*, 9 January: retrieved 2 June 2008, from http://www.smh.com.au/news/opinion/fat-divide-between-classes/2007/01/08/1168104921042.html

Deleuze, G. (1992) 'Postscript on the societies of control', *October*, 59: 3–7.

Deleuze, G. (2000) *Foucault*, trans. S. Hand, Minneapolis: The University of Minnesota Press.

Department of Consumer and Employment Protection, Government of Western Australia (2008) 'Reversing the global wave of childhood obesity', *Better Trading*, 6: retrieved 20 June 2008, from http://www.docep.wa.gov.au/Consumer-Protection/Content/bettertrading/Issue/article_1.html

Devechi, S., Gülbayrak, C., Oğuzöncül, A. and Açik, Y. (2004) 'The prevalence of obesity in police officers admitting to the outpatient department of a security department health office in Elazığ', *F.Ü. Sağlık Bil*, 18(4): 223–8.

Gard, M. and Wright, J. (2005) *The Obesity Epidemic*, London: Routledge.

Hagan, T. (2008) 'Fight against obesity early: parents need to shape up', *The Observer*, 10 May: retrieved 10 May 2008, from http://www.theobserver.ca/ArticleDisplay.aspx?e=983678

Halse, C. (2006) 'Writing/reading a life: the rhetorical practice of autobiography', *Auto/biography*, 14(2): 95–115.

Halse, C., Honey, A. and Boughtwood, D. (2007) 'The paradox of virtue: (re)thinking deviance, anorexia and schooling', *Gender and Education*, 19(2): 219–35.

Hunter, M. (2008) 'Surgeon general lauds family weight-loss program', *The Times-Picayune*, 8 May: retrieved 8 May 2008, from http://www.nola.com/news/index.ssf/2008/05/ymca_family_weightloss_program.html%20Accessed%2010%20May%202008

Ironside, R. (2008) 'Call for height and weight restrictions for police', *Courier Mail*, 18 May: retrieved 1 June 2008, from http://www.news.com.au/courier-mail/story/0,23739,23718612-952,00.html

James, P.T., Leach, R., Kalamara, E. and Shayeghi, M. (2001) 'The worldwide obesity epidemic', *Obesity Research*, 9: 228–33.

McDowell, D.L. (2008) 'Kids in the kitchen: Junior League starts delicious fight against childhood obesity', *The Daily News Journal*, April 29: retrieved 12 May 2008, from http://dnj.midsouthnews.com/apps/pbcs.dll/article?AID=/20080429/LIFESTYLE/804290304/1024%20Accessed%2010%20May%202008

Mayo Foundation for Medical Education and Research (MFMER) (2006) *Childhood Obesity: make weight loss a family affair*, retrieved 17 May 2008, from www.mayoclinic.com/health/childhood-obesity/FL0005

No Author (2002) *Family Loses Custody of Overweight Girl*, retrieved 15 May 2008, from http://www.apfn.org/apfn/overweight.htm

No Author (2006a) 'Obesity blame game', *Journal of the Diabetes Association*, 3(3): 20.

No Author (2006b) 'Obesity epidemic calls for whole of society solutions', *The Age*, 5 September: retrieved 5 January 2008, from http://tertiary.theage.com.au/bmentry_view.asp?intid=37

No Author (2006c) 'Pie eating championship goes slimline', *The Guardian*, 23 November: retrieved 2 January 2008, from http://www.guardian.co.uk/uk/2006/nov/23/foodanddrink

No Author (2006d) 'Thin can be fat inside', *Sydney Morning Herald*, 13 December: 3.

No Author (2007a) 'Legislators in Florida tackle childhood obesity', weblog post, *My Overweight Child*, 11 April: retrieved 15 May 2008, from http://www.myoverweightchild.com/blog/2007/04/legislators-in-florida-tackle-childhood.html

No Author (2007b) 'PE added to NCLB', weblog post, *My Overweight Child*: retrieved 15 May 2008, from http://www.myoverweightchild.com/blog/index.html

No Author (2008a) *My Overweight Child*, weblog: retrieved 15 May 2008, from http://www.myoverweightchild.com/blog/index.html

No Author (2008b) 'New North Carolina initiative addresses physical activity', weblog post, *My Overweight Child*, 30 March: retrieved 15 May 2008, from http://www.myoverweightchild.com/blog/2008/03/new-north-carolina-initiative-addresses.html

No Author (2008c) 'State passes ban on trans-fats', weblog, *My Overweight Child*, 30 April: retrieved 15 May 2008, from http://www.myoverweightchild.com/blog/index.html

Oliver, J.E. (2005) *Fat Politics: The Real Story Behind America's Obesity Epidemic*, Oxford and New York: Oxford University Press.

Perritt, H. (2002) *Americans with Disabilities Act Handbook*, New York: Aspen Publishers.

Prioietto, J. and Baur, L. (2004) 'The management of obesity', *The Medical Journal of Australia*, 180: 474—80:retrieved 15 May 2008, fromhttp://www.mja.com.au/public/issues/180_09_030504/pro10445_fm.html

Rabinow, P. and Rose, N. (2003) *Thoughts on the Concept of Biopower Today*: Retrieved 30 June 2008, from http://www.lse.ac.uk/collections/sociology/pdf/RabinowandRose-BiopowerToday03.pdf

Rawls, J. (1971/1999) *A Theory of Justice*, Cambridge, Massachusetts: Belknap Press of Harvard University Press.

Roehling, M.V. (1999) 'Weight-based discrimination in employment: psychological and legal aspects', *Personnel Psychology*, 52(4): 969–1016.

Rose, N. (1999) *Powers of Freedom: Reframing Political Thought*, Cambridge, Mass: Cambridge University Press.

Rose, N. and Novas, C. (2003) 'Biological Citizenship', in A. Ong and S. Collier (eds) *Global Anthropology*, London: Blackwell.

Smith, A. (2008) 'Obesity crisis calls for more heavy-duty ambulances', *Sydney Morning Herald*, 11 February: retrieved 1 June 2008, from http://www.smh.com.au/news/national/obesity-crisis-calls-for-more-heavyduty-ambulances/2008/02/10/1202578600937.html

Streib, L. (2007) 'World's fattest countries', *Forbes Magazine*, 2 August: retrieved 13 May 2008, from http://www.forbes.com/2007/02/07/worlds-fattest-countries-forbeslife-cx_ls_0208worldfat.html

Subcommittee on Military Weight Management, and Committee on Military Nutrition Research (2004) *Weight Management: State of the Science and Opportunities for Military Programs*, Washington: National Academies Press.

The Centre for Consumer Freedom (2008) *About Us*, retrieved 11 May 2008, from http://www.consumerfreedom.com/about.cfm.

Trust for America's Health (2007) *F as in Fat: How Obesity Policies are Failing in America*, retrieved 2 January, from http://healthyamericans.org/reports/obesity2006/

Turner, B. (1994) 'General Commentary', in B. Turner and P. Hamilton (eds) *Citizenship: Critical Concepts*, vol. 1, New York: Routledge.

Uhlmann, C. (2006) 'Obesity epidemic costing Australia $3 billion a year', on *The World Today [radio program]*, ABC Local Radio, 18 October.

5 Doctor's Orders
Diagnosis, Medical Authority and the Exploitation of the Fat Body

Annemarie Jutel

INTRODUCTION

Medicine is pivotal in the discussion of overweight and obesity. Condemnation of overweight hinges on the premise that it is a disease that puts individuals at risk and renders populations vulnerable. Yet ironically, less than a century ago, plumpness was lauded as healthy, and slenderness a cause for concern. Medical textbooks were more likely to be preoccupied by the risk of underweight than of fatness. In 1929, J.P. MacLaren recommended to doctors undertaking medical insurance examinations that 'generally speaking, a moderate accumulation of fat up to the age of 40 or 45 is good,' and, he explained, 'if the subject has a broad chest, muscular frame, good digestion and circulation and active habits, his chances of longevity are distinctly good' (MacLaren 1929: 192). At odds with contemporary beliefs, MacLaren described the overweight youth as a much lower risk than the underweight to the potential insurer.

Weight on its own, outside of any health education initiative, cultural pressure or unexpected fluctuation, is unlikely to be perceived as illness by a heavy person. Illness might include shortness of breath, unusual swelling in the feet, or other forms of distress, but is unlikely to include measurement. I speak of illness in contrast to disease, that on the other hand, is a discrete entity, defined and scoped by the medical institution. Many people are heavy and feel no physical or social distress and hence would have no cause to consider themselves ill. As Eisenberg and Kleinman (1980: 13) point out, '[a] visit to the doctor is more likely when disease is present, but it is essential to understand that contracting a disease, feeling ill and being a patient are overlapping but not co-extensive states'.

Nonetheless, plumpness has been referred to as a problematic condition for centuries. Hippocrates (1978) made reference to an increase in mortality in fat people as compared to thin people. In contradistinction, preoccupation with overweight, and even the concept itself, are relatively recent. I will argue in this chapter that the medical and lay communities consider overweight—measured deviation from what is considered to be normal weight—to be a disease. This consideration is at the base of exploitative commercial practices that fuel the idea that there is an epidemic of overweight. To present this argument, I will first introduce the evidence that supports my assertion that there has been a change in the past decade in the way that the medical literature has approached overweight as a clinical entity. Secondly, I will point out the convergence of conditions that have led to the consideration of overweight as disease rather than as measurement. Finally, I will demonstrate how the disease label provides an efficient and effective mechanism to exploit lay fear of fat and obesity for commercial ends. I will make this demonstration explicit through Zola's (1983) tenets of medicalization that posit that medicine exerts political power through its status as 'repository of truth' in contemporary society.

THE EMERGENCE OF OVERWEIGHT AS A DISEASE ENTITY

Diagnosis, or the identification of the presence of a disease, is pivotal in how medicine exerts social control. It legitimizes and normalizes, providing the boundaries for what is acceptable, as well as identifying what is problematic, and in need of redress. *Giving the name* is often the starting point for social labellers and is a *language of medicine* (Brown 1995). Diagnosis formalizes conditions that either individual or society identifies as problematic.

Diagnosis can also be enabling, providing a trajectory of treatment, prognosis and possibly prevention, and placing the patient in the conceptual company of others with the same affliction. Formal diagnoses organize symptoms into meaningful concepts. The urinary frequency becomes diabetes; the rash, lupus; and the cough, bronchitis. Whilst the diagnosis is not necessarily welcome, it nonetheless provides a structure for anticipating what will happen next and what measures to take to remedy or at least, palliate the condition.

But, diagnosis also controls, compelling the patient to become obedient to a new set of normative obligations including incapacity and therapeutic compliance, that can even be mandated, in the case of some diagnoses. Coughing—a symptom—might lead an individual to cover her mouth, and consult a doctor, whereas active tuberculosis or pertussis—diagnoses both—result in enforced respiratory isolation and mandatory reporting to health authorities. Diagnosis affects outcomes. As Hamilton and colleagues have revealed, giving a particular disease label, when a range of options is available may result in a different prognosis (Hamilton Campos and Creed 1996). Haynes and colleagues (1978) reported that labelling patients hypertensive, for example, increased absenteeism from work.

Many factors influence what will receive disease status. Technical knowledge, social values, the nature of the biological condition and institutionalized processes all contribute to what may receive a disease label.

For example, from the point of view of the World Health Organization or an insurance company rigid classification determines what can be counted statistically as disease or be deemed worthy of financial reimbursement for treatment. But the classification of diseases is fluid. Some diseases have not yet been discovered, others have not been named, and again others are not at this time considered diseases, although they may be so considered in other times or contexts. New diseases emerge while others fade into oblivion. Chlorosis, for example, an antique affliction, with a peak in prevalence in the nineteenth century and presumed today to be an iron-deficiency anaemia, has not been reported since the 1930s. Its disappearance is attributed by some to improved prophylactic measures and diagnostic skills, by others to improved social and hygienic conditions (Guggenheim 1995).

On the other hand, Alzheimer's disease was unknown until 1907. Its 'discovery' was made possible by the introduction of new laboratory techniques that enabled its differentiation from other forms of dementia and its description as a new complex clinicopathologic entity (Amaducci et al. 1986). This discovery does not reflect a new neurological process; rather new diagnostic tools capable of categorising what might previously have been considered an inevitable sign of normal aging. Medical science's ability to see and classify has changed. As the knowledge base changes, so too do the notions of what constitutes health and illness as well as what individuals are willing to endure without remedy or palliation.

Diseases also reflect social concern. For example, when Dr Cartwright (1981: 320) wrote his 1851 treatise on the 'diseases of Negroes' he described 'drapetomania', or 'the disease causing slaves to run away': an example of a condition that contemporary critics see firmly founded in social values, rather than in medicine or biology. More recently, in 1994, the American Psychiatric Association discarded the term 'homosexuality' from the *Diagnostic and Statistical Manual of Mental Disorders*, reflecting a change in the consideration of sexuality (Mendelson 2003). A contemporary example is the term 'excited delirium', in wide use by medical examiners to describe clinical manifestations resulting from presumed medical illness or substance abuse, necessitating forcible restraint, and often resulting in death (Channa Perera and Pollanen 2006; Pacquette 2003). Yet, one can argue that this diagnosis is not a medical condition, rather a mechanism for transferring the responsibility for death to a pathophysiological entity rather than to police brutality in the presence of difficult behaviours.

Historically, overweight has not always been treated as if it were a disease, but I argue in this chapter, that overweight gained disease status at the end of the twentieth century. I maintain that this transformation of the way that weight is considered by the medical community facilitates commercial claims about products targeting plump individuals. Note that I am not here speaking of obesity, that has its own classificatory framework, and definitions, and that merits its own analysis; rather I write about overweight, a term that semantically refers to any amount of weight that is in excess of a particular standard.

A review of medical publications from 1964 to 2004, results of which I have published elsewhere (Jutel 2006) demonstrates a change in the language used to discuss overweight. Where the word overweight figured more prominently in titles of medical articles to refer to a sign or symptom, today, the word appears more frequently to describe a condition with its own set of risk factors, typologies, outcomes, treatment and prevention, all suggestive of overweight-as-disease. For example, earlier references would be predominantly to 'overweight persons', 'overweight in an obesity clinic', or 'overweight and hypertension' where the term is used as an adjective, or to describe a symptom, often subordinated to another condition. There is a distinct trend in recent years to refer to overweight as a disease on its own. This can be found in wording such as 'identification, evaluation and treatment of overweight', 'the epidemic of overweight', 'risk factors for overweight', or by using the word in a non-subordinate list of other recognized diagnoses.

Any one of a number of documents, often generated by authoritative organizations such as health ministries and their equivalents, mirror this general transformation in word use, using the language normally reserved for diseases to refer to overweight. For example, *Clinical Guidelines on the identification, evaluation, and treatment of overweight and obesity in adults*, by the National Institutes of Health (NIH) (1998) speaks of *treatment* and *prevention* of overweight, and are concerned with reducing its *prevalence*. The Centre for Disease Control (CDC) (2005) in its document 'Diseases and Conditions' includes overweight and provides links to teaching documents that explain the prevalence of overweight has increased to 'epidemic proportions'. By placing overweight as an object of epidemiological study, and using the language associated with the study of disease, the CDC confirms again the consideration of overweight as disease. Similarly, Australia, Great Britain, France, the United States, Canada, New Zealand and many other countries have an array of position papers, clinical guidelines and expert task force reports on the 'prevention' and 'treatment' of overweight (Jutel 2001).

THE CONVERGENCE OF CONDITIONS

A number of factors together combine to create the context in which overweight has come to be treated as a disease, rather than just a measurement. Firstly, an important principle that buttresses the pathologizing of overweight is the assumption that the appearance of the body reveals the nature of the individual; whether this be their moral or a physical nature, it is assumed to be observed externally by a person's form. A second fundamental factor in this transformation of overweight from statistical deviance to disease is the generalized ability to measure fatness. In the scientific-based model, measurement is perceived to be an objective means of assessment, and scales thus become more reliable than individuals in establishing the truth. Thirdly, the tenets of evidence-based medicine (EBM) privilege quantitative measurement. The hierarchies of knowledge recognized by EBM place great importance on statistical analysis; a quantifiable category such as weight slots in this framework most harmoniously.

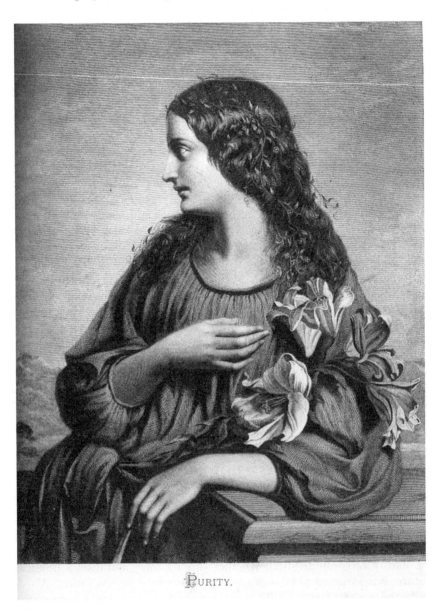

PURITY.

Figure 5.1   Purity

And finally, the rhetoric of medicine serves an important role in the marketing of products and services that, in turn, have a powerful participatory interest in promoting overweight as a disease.

Appearance Reveals Health

Writings as early as the New Testament—where the Virgin Mary's purity was associated with a spotless mirror, thus aligning perfection of image and of character—provide evidence of the longevity of assumptions about appearance confering insights to a person's true nature. Books from the Renaissance; assumed that beauty reflected goodness ugliness, evil. For example, Baldessare Castiglione (1561/1948: 309) wrote: '[v]ery seldom [doth] an ill soule dwell in a beautifull bodie. And therefore is the outwarde beautie a true signe of the inwarde goodnesse'. Francis Bacon (1664: 245–6) echoed these ideas 100 years later when he asserted: '[d]eformed persons are commonly even with Nature, for as nature hath done ill by them, so do they by Nature, being for the most part (as the Scripture saith) *Void of natural Affection*'. The back of Leonardo da Vinci's portrait, *Ginevra de'Benci* carries the inscription: 'Beauty Adorns Virtue' (Brown 2001). In folk tales, heroes and heroines are either beautiful or will so become (Cinderella, Rapunzel, the Frog Prince), and villains are ugly. Frequently, pictures are used by publishers to illustrate character traits, as indicated in Figure 5.1.

By the end of the nineteenth century, however, the inner fibre captured in appearance was no longer virtue, but health. References to good health pervaded discussions of beauty. In 1896, Ayer advocated its Sarsaparilla as a blood cleanser: 'Beauty begins in the blood' and reports that 'Beauty is blood deep, not "skin deep"' (Ayer's Sarsaparilla 1896: 115). In the same magazine, The California Fig Syrup Company (1896: 115) reminded readers that 'one of the greatest factors in producing a clear, clean skin and therefore a perfect complexion, is the use of Syrup of Figs'. And the Pabst Brewing Company spoke of a young mother 'flushed with perfect health' after consuming Pabst Malt Extract, the 'best' tonic (Pabst Brewing Company, 1897: 115). Later, Andrews Liver Salts (a laxative) proposed 'inner cleanliness' as a beauty treatment. 'Andrews settles the stomach, corrects acidity . . . thus helping to clear up the spots due to digestive disturbance' (Andrew's Liver Salts 1941: 245) (see Figure 5.2).

This link between health and beauty is neither simply historical, nor limited to lay perspectives and advertising. How an individual looks when he or she presents for medical consultation is likely to have a strong influence on the diagnostic process. For example, Pat Croskerry (2002), writing on medical education, points out the important role that visual assessment plays in clinical reasoning; it establishes pattern recognition that sets the frame for the clinical work-up. This is understandable, and in many ways unproblematic. Visual cues, such as pallor, jaundice, pupil reactivity, swelling, and alopecia and so on are fundamental to diagnosis. However, as

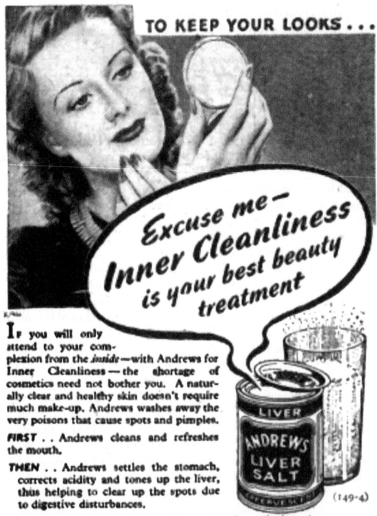

Figure 5.2   Andrews Liver Salt.

Stafford and colleagues (Stafford, La Puma and Schiedermayer 1989) caution, what clinicians see is also influenced by their perceptual preferences
and can play out dangerously in medical judgments about the 'abnormal'.
There is a standard of homogeneity, write Stafford et al., that governs how
medical professionals respond to patients, how the law protects patient
rights and what defines medical priorities.

Zola's (1983) discussion of medicalization asserts that medicine practices under what it, and society at large, considers to be noble neutrality and objectivity, justification for its role as repository of truth. Yet, cultural values are just as deeply ingrained in medicine as they are in other settings and to presume a greater objectivity of the medical eye is to overlook the fact that, 'there is no guarantee that merely doing the job of "healing" frees one from examining the context within that it is carried out' (p. 272).

Stafford and her colleagues (Stafford et al. 1989: 214) explain, '[t]he unstated perceptual norm that governs our reactions to patients is predicated on a symmetrical and minimalist conception of beauty'. They maintain that physiology, ethics and aesthetics attempted historically, and continue to attempt to capture the symmetry of beauty or of good. 'Good' numbers, like beautiful things, reflect a kind of perfection in geometry or of form that have implications for the notion of what it means to be healthy. Weighing the body is one important way for determining this symmetry and normality.

Corpulence is Quantified

Nineteenth century medical dictionaries highlight the qualitative, rather than quantitative, nature of adiposity. Obesity was, according to Herrick (1889: 272), in *A Reference Handbook of the Medical Sciences*, 'an increased bulk of the body, beyond what is sightly and healthy', and to Thomas (1891: 458), 'corpulence; fatness or grossness of the body . . . characterized by an excessive development of the adipose tissue'. That these descriptions should be qualitative is not surprising, given that scales were not necessarily readily available to the doctor. These were expensive tools that did not become prevalent until well into the twentieth century.

Historian Peter Stearns (1997) related that weight was not even part of medical record keeping until the late nineteenth century. Whilst the New England Hospital for Women and Children had pre-printed forms with spaces for pulse, temperature, respiratory rate and weight, the space for weight alone was often left blank. Scales were not necessarily part of the doctor's armoury. At the end of the nineteenth century, in presenting the 'Reliance Weighing Machine' in their 'Notes and Short Comment' section, the Lancet (1897: 1316) editors write that 'hitherto, these personal weighing machines have taken up too much room in a consulting room and the expense has been too great'. Whilst they may not have previously been part of the doctor's assessment tools, the importance of weighing undoubtedly grew with their availability, as well as with the primacy accorded to concepts of evidence in medicine. Public scales began to spread from 1891 onwards and scales for private homes first hit the market in 1913 (Stearns 1997).

Instruments of Precision

The transformation of obesity into a measurable state may have taken place at the beginning of the twentieth century, but this transformation did not 'take' immediately in the medical community. Whilst measurement of the body was part of a general endeavour to establish rules about the nature of mankind and of sub-groups within the species,[1] using measurement for the assessment of physical health, on the other hand, was not as prevalent. The earliest height and weight tables actually emerged from actuarial rather than medical research. The Medico–Actuarial society compiled the content of 812,221 client 'build cards', to identify actual and expected deaths of, and by extension, financial risk presented by, policy owners of varying weights (Joint Committee 1913).

These height/weight charts, designed to reply to the economic motive of insurance selection, were assimilated by the medical community, though initially with resistance. 'No weight table is sufficient by itself to base an estimate of the ideal state', wrote William Christie in 1927. 'Standard tables that show the average for men and women of our race at any given age and height are fallacious, because no allowance is made for the distinctions of personal physique, nor consideration given to obvious rolls of fat' (Christie 1927: 23). Dr Jean Leray, in his 1931 analysis of plumpness[2] and obesity expressed scepticism about tables, despite devoting a number of pages to the different formulas and tables that could be used to identify the perfect healthy weight. Leray referred to these calculations as being of 'theoretical interest' only, and instead used Leven's practice of defining safe body weight as the average weight a person in good health maintains over a number of years (Leray 1931). Leray argued that the correct weight for an individual could not be determined by standardized table.

On the other hand, Royal Copeland (1922), a prolific writer on the subject of obesity, made no qualms about using the 1913 Medico–Actuarial tables. It is worth noting that his *Overweight? guard your health* was a trade book, and perhaps sought a short cut to self-diagnosis, an important tool in product marketing as we will see over-leaf. Height and weight charts did however become standard fixtures in medical textbooks, and as late as 1940, Dr Hugo Rony's (1940) medical textbook *Obesity and Leanness* still relied upon the 1913 actuarial studies.

Scales became part of the trend towards, as Rosenberg (2002) describes, 'instruments of precision', that emerged in the late nineteenth century. These apparatuses, including microscopes, thermometers, and later manometers, radiology equipment, electrocardiogram machines, offered objective mechanisms for capturing, standardizing and monitoring disease. Being able to express results in standardized units enabled, Rosenberg argues, disease to be 'operationally understood and described. It was measured in units, represented in the visible forms of curves or continuous tracings' (p. 244). This standardisation and measurability form the base both of contemporary diagnosis, epidemiology and evidence-based medicine (EBM) that produces and reproduces overweight as a disease entity.

Evidence-based medicine, that has evolved in the last decades of the twentieth century, promotes particular forms of therapeutic knowledge. It is a practice developed in a positivist framework that emerged from a series of lectures by epidemiologist, Archie Cochrane who argued that clinical decisions were too-often based on inadequate or dubious information, and that the medical profession should continuously evaluate the knowledge base upon that it made its decisions (Ashcroft 2004).

Evidence-based practice has since pervaded medical and allied health practice, and is the cornerstone to strategic plans and competency frameworks in medicine, nursing and other allied health fields. Proponents, such as David Sackett and colleagues (Sackett Straus Richardson Rosenberg and Haynes 2000) have published how-to guides to practicing and teaching EBM. Importantly it, as other textbooks (see, for example, Courtney 2005; DiCenso Guyatt and Ciliska 2005; Straus Richardson Glasziou and Haynes 2005) on evidence in health practice, ranks statistical (measurable/quantifiable) knowledge well above other forms. The hierarchical approach to knowledge situates systematic review and randomized controlled trials at the highest level of evidence, in front of non-randomized, case reports and case series.

What this does, however, is to privilege the tenets of experimental knowledge that itself is based upon values that enable standardisation. This requires variability to be defined, populations discerned, results compared and similarities to the patient established by clinicians. Implicit, therefore, in the research-based or experimental model is the quantification of cause and effect, and the measurement of, and focus on, in this case, body weight. In Sackett's personal introduction to the book he co-authors (Sackett et al. 2000) he expresses his interest in, and motivation to, implement evidence-based medicine as coming from a chance stint performing surveys of cardiovascular disease. He writes that it occurred to him that 'epidemiology and biostatistics could be made as relevant to clinical medicine as . . . research into the tubular transport of amino acids'. The purpose of this article is not to dispute this approach, although others have done so vigorously (see, for example, Holmes Murray Perron and Rail 2006; Morse 2006; Rolfe 2005). It is rather to show that an evidence-based framework of clinical practice contributes strongly to shifting the quantifiable category of overweight towards disease status.

With the ability to quantify corpulence comes the potential to track its distribution, prevalence and correlates. In turn, this allows a description of normality and a delineation of the bounds of normal build, which subsequently naturalizes concepts of difference and deviance. Numbers enable clinicians practicing in an evidence-based framework to rely upon information that is well placed in the information hierarchy. Information presented by the patient sits in a subordinated position on the hierarchy. It is assumed by science to be subjective and contaminated by patients' investments in their own lifestyles; information may be embellished, distorted or misrepresented. On the other hand, the scales don't lie. Furthermore, a strong antifat stigma adds to the negative perception of patient report. For example, a study of physicians' automatic response to their obese patients found they thought these patients were bad and lazy (Hebl and Xu 2001). Crandall (1994) also found that health professionals thought heavy people were less reliable and trustworthy than thin. Scales, in this context and with these belief systems, would be perceived to provide a more valuable report.

Historian Hillel Schwartz (1986: 147) in his cultural history of diets argued, 'the body when weighed told the truth about the self. Once gluttony had been linked to fatness and fatness to heaviness, heaviness had still to be regularly identified by numbers on a scale, rather than by vague and subjective sensations'. As Foucault (1963) wrote in his history of the clinic, the medical gaze saw the patient as a barrier to the truth. 'In order to know the truth of the pathological fact, the doctor must abstract the patient . . . the medical gaze . . . [addresses] all that which is visible in illness, but starting from the patient, who hides that which is visible by showing it' (Foucault 1963: 8, my translation). In the clinical assessment, the patient's story is thus an obstruction to the clinician's discovery of the facts of the illness.

An example of silencing the patient can be seen in the National Institutes of Health (NIH) (1998) *Clinical Guidelines on the Identification, Evaluation and Treatment of Overweight and Obesity in Adults: The Evidence Report*. This document is considered a gold standard of evidence for the management of overweight by American and Western medical institutions in the context of evidencebased medicine. It makes treatment recommendations on the basis of extensive review of empirical studies. The treatment recommendations are summarized in an algorithm (see Figure 5.3). This schematic flow chart prompts doctors with respect to the appropriate actions to take to determine if a patient has a weight problem. However, said actions are purely measurementbased. The patient should be, according to these instructions, weighed and measured, but not interviewed. The only suggestion that a patient might have information to offer doctors assess his or her health is subordinated by the grammatical use of the conditional: patient input 'may' be helpful.

The result of this is to allow scales to dictate wellness and create a convenient mechanism for understanding corpulence. Because scales are no longer the preserve of the doctor, and are prevalent in most households, they enable self-diagnosis, and generate an exploitable condition, fruitful to the economic interest of a range of product and service providers, as we will see below.

Medicalization and the Exploitation of the Disease Label

I started this chapter by pointing out how diagnoses reflected the anxieties of a particular society at a particular time in the presence of technological tools enabling their definition. Perhaps we can see a circular relationship here. On the one hand, overweight as a diagnosis reflects the concern of a society that believes normative appearance to be predictive of health. On

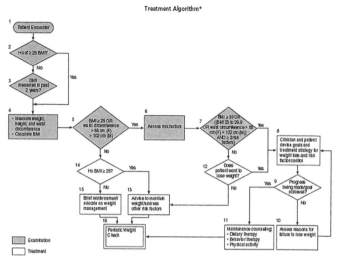

Figure 5.3   Algorithm.

the other, however, the power of medicine as an institution reproduces this anxiety as it validates and provides scientific credibility to the concern.

Diagnosis is pivotal in the way that medicine exerts its social control. It legitimizes that which either individual or society identify as problematic. In the sixteenth century, it was a psychiatrist who argued that witches should not be burned. They were insane, he argued, rather than possessed by the devil (Gevitz 2000). As mentioned above, homosexuality has variously been defined as moral decadence, biological illness, or a normal practice within the continuum of human sexuality; medicine, notably the American Psychiatric Association's *Diagnostic and Statistic Manual (DSM)*, has variably included and removed homosexuality as a clinical entity, typifying its changing social status (Mendelson 2003).

But medicine also serves to reproduce values through its rhetoric and endorsement. Zola coined the term 'medicalization' in the late 1960s, describing it as the means by which medicine's influence and jurisdiction expands to create a distinct political form of social control, usually to the detriment of any one of a number of vulnerable populations (Zola 1986). The discourses of medicine, its language and rhetoric, play an important role in extending its moral authority. 'There is an aura of objectivity', writes Zola, 'that surrounds not only medicine but its pronouncements' (p. 272). Thus, products that appear to respond to a medical need, whose promotion is couched in medicalese, or are supported by medical research, gain purchase in the popular psyche.

Helping people to consider themselves ill or at risk of illness provides a platform for piggybacking commercial interests onto medical authority. And, creating a disease category out of a self-identifiable statistical deviation such as weight enables the commercial exploitation of those so afflicted. Self-assessment tools generate significant consumer interest (McEntee 2003). Those conditions that can easily be diagnosed by a consumer without medical intervention are particularly attractive to industry. For example, Body Mass Index (BMI) calculators are popular features on pharmaceutical weight loss medications sites, as the Abbott Laboratories' promotion of sibutramine hydrochloride monohydrate, or Meridia (Abbot Laboratories 2007). But the weight loss industry extends well beyond the pharmaceutical companies alone and plays an important role in the generation and promulgation of the diagnosis of overweight.

The number of industries who stand to benefit from the belief that overweight is disease is strong, and results in significant lobbying and product promotion based on the disease label (Oliver 2006). Weight reduction, muscle tone and body shape are exceptionally strong markers of 'health' to consumers (Spitzack 1990). The gym, diet, self-help, cosmetic, pharmaceutical and many other industries all have a financial stake in ensuring that people see their weight as problematic from a medical point of view (Jutel and Buetow 2007).

Conrad (2005) has referred to the commercial interests as an important vehicle for medicalization. Examples of an implied medical endorsement for products and services are prevalent in advertising strategies, particularly in what Dixon and Banwell (2004) refer to as a 'diets-making complex', or a vehicle, often exploitative, for the dominance of health considerations in all facets of dietary discourse. By transferring such information to the consumer, there is an implied recognition of lay knowledge of health risk, buttressed by authoritative medical discourse and language that draw the individual into a closed circle of virtuous consumers who focus on important evidence-based truths.

The diet industry, but also others that stand to benefit from belief in overweight-as-disease use this abundantly. For example, milk advertisements quote model Elizabeth Hurley saying: 'I want to look great and milk helps. *Studies suggest* [italics mine] that people who drink milk regularly tend to weigh less and have less body fat than those who don't' (2424Milk 2006); Les Mills Gym publishes press releases from the World Health Organization to promote weight loss programmes (Les Mills 2006); and Schwinn Bicycles (Schwinn Fitness 2006) points out that 'being overweight can contribute to an increased risk in heart attack, diabetes, high blood pressure and other *life threatening illnesses* [italics mine]'. They also refer to *research* [italics mine] that reassures us we don't have to train too hard to remove these risk factors. Once the sales pitch is justified by the austere and respected guardian of Western culture—medical authority, the product has more clout and less frivolity. The consumer becomes a virtuous and docile subject as she complies through her purchasing decisions.

Overweight, like Adult Attention Deficit Hyperactivity Disorder (ADHD), Erectile Dysfunction and pregnancy, is a condition that, once defined as medical, exposes those who experience them to risks that are not present prior to such definition. A notable component of that risk results from the commercial target they have become, and the mongering of products that may ensue. But actually mongering the disease label, or encouraging individuals to believe themselves either sick or at risk of so becoming, is of growing concern to critical clinicians, advocates, and lay people (Moynihan and Henry 2006). Disease mongering creates a belief in and promotion of conditions for which clinical attention may cause more harm than benefit. Whether it be the pharmaceutical industry, peddling sibutramine or orlistat (known by the trade names of Reductil and Xenical); the media, promoting its diet or lifestyle modification reality shows (*Biggest Loser, Honey We're Killing the Kids*); the diet industry (Weight Watchers, Jenny Craig); the gym and fitness industry or many others, there is a vast array of commercial interests primed to wage battle, purportedly for the health of the nation, whilst cheerfully amassing the spoils of their continual and repeated victories for their shareholders; and many protect their interests through their lobbying and consultative role to health agencies. Australia's weight loss policy paper *Acting on Australia's Weight,* for example, uses the weight loss industry as a key player in the education for the prevention of overweight, which it identifies as an area for strategic action. The panel actually hands a portion of the responsibility for the prevention of overweight directly to this private industry player who stands to make significant financial gains from suggesting that weights should be monitored, controlled, and possibly reduced (Jutel 2001).

The victory is not thinness, it is the undying belief in overweight-as-disease. As long as mongerers of overweight, bolstered by medicine's implied endorsement, can continue to convince individuals to hold to the belief that plumpness attests to self-induced disease, they can reap certain benefit, selling their fitness programmes; dietary supplements; self-help guides; television shows; metabolism boosters; diet pills; cellulite busters; weight machines; diet plans; low-fat, high-protein, low-GI food stuffs; and so on.

CONCLUSION

Ivan Illich (1976: 104), in his scathing seminal work on the medicalization of the human existence, wrote that 'disease always intensifies stress, defines incapacity, imposes inactivity, and focuses apprehension on non-recovery, on uncertainty, and on one's dependence upon future medical findings'. He continues, '[o]nce a society organizes for a preventative disease-hunt, it gives epidemic proportions to diagnosis. This ultimate triumph of therapeutic culture turns the independence of the average healthy person into an intolerable form of deviance'. These words are particularly poignant when we reflect upon contemporary Western culture's focus on the slender body.

Not only does overweight-as-disease transform independence into deviance, the simplicity of its diagnostic work-up (simply step on the scales) enables dangerous constraints. Weight is only a number, but a very powerful one. Just as the perfect hourglass figure might have been 34–23–35, or the perfect size six, today's standards of perfection are captured in BMI, health policy, medical management and product sales.

Again, Illich (1976: 53): '[m]edicine is a moral enterprise, and therefore inevitably gives content to good and evil. In every society, medicine, like law and religion, defines what is normal, proper or desirable'. Overweight-as-disease uses detached objective numbers without regard to important principles about populations and individuals. It disenfranchises the individual as it privileges measurement over lived experience, validates presumed behaviours and reveals moral flaws.

But overweight-as-disease is a marketer's ploy made in heaven. Here we have a self-diagnosable condition that engenders a population-wide preoccupation with self-surveillance, treatment, prevention and cure. Monitoring is internalized; compliance to 'healthy' practices denotes virtue. The individual body is rendered docile by the medicalization of its management by commercial entities. As with the panopticon, the doctor need not be present to ensure compliance: the individual, with scales and ruler can diagnose overweight. A smorgasbord of web sites allows consumers to plug in numbers and push the button for instant BMI calculations (General Mills 2008; Jenny Craig 2008; Total Gym 2008). Once measured, it doesn't take a doctor to position the number within or outside of the acceptable standard,[3] or to decide the range of interventions to take.

It is hard to appreciate the cultural content of a diagnosis that emerges from a contemporary context. As members of the society that suffers the anxiety over weight that results from its creation as disease, we don't have the same critical distance as we have with respect to hysteria or, say onanism. Most readers of this chapter will likely be aware of their body size and firmness, concerned if it increases, ostracized if they are large, and possibly even inclined to say 'make that trim milk please' when they have the option. Overweight is an excellent illustration of the influence of culture on diagnostic categories, and similarly of the important role that diagnosis plays in the production and reproduction of cultural values.

NOTES

1. The Body Mass Index, used today as an index of overweight and obesity, was devised by Adolphe Quetelet (1871) and was motivated by the religious incentive of discovering the presence of God's rules on earth.
2. It is interesting to note that the original French title of this book, *Embonpoint et obesité* flags an important conceptual shift. Embonpoint, translated here as 'plumpness' has as its etymological source 'en bon point' or 'en bon état' meaning being in good health, or looking well. Its modern

meaning, and indeed, its meaning at the time of Leray's writing, however, is to be plump.

3. The fact that population statistics are being used indiscriminately without regard to cultural group, and without identification of the sample group from which normative standards were derived, is neglected by both marketer, doctor and individual.

REFERENCES

2424milk (2006) *Milk Your Diet. Lose Weight!*, retrieved 14 July 2006, from http://2424milk.com/index.htm

Abbot Laboratories (2007) *Personal Weight Assessment*, retrieved 4 February 2007, from http://www.meridia.net/dsp_consumer_bmi.cfm

Amaducci, L.A., Rocca, W.A. and Schoenberg, B.S. (1986) 'Origin of the distinction between Alzheimer's disease and senile dementia: how history can clarify nosology', *Neurology*, 36: 1497–9.

Andrew's Liver Salts (1941) 'Inner cleanliness', *Woman's Weekly*, 23 August: 245.

Ashcroft, R.E. (2004) 'Current epistemological problems in evidence based medicine', *Journal of Medical Ethics*, 30: 131–5.

Ayer's Sarsaparilla (1896) 'Beauty begins in the blood'. *Godey's Magazine.*

Bacon, F. (1664) *Essayes and Counsels, Civil and Moral*, London: Thomas Palmer.

Bandura, A., Adams, N.E., Hardy, A.B. and Howells, G.N. (1980) 'Tests of the generality of self-efficacy theory', *Cognitive Therapy and Research*, 4:39–66.

Brown, D.A. (2001) *Virtue and Beauty*, Princeton, NJ: Princeton University Press.

Brown, P. (1995) 'Naming and framing: the social construction of diagnosis and illness', *Journal of Health and Social Behavior*, Spec No.: 34–52.

California Fig Company (1986) 'Syrup of Figs', *Godey's*. January: back cover.

Cartwright, S. (1981) 'Report of the Diseases and Physical Peculiarities of the Negro Race', in A. Caplan, H.T. Englehardt and J. McCartney (eds) *Concepts of Health and Disease*. Reading, MA: Addison-Wesley Publishing Company.

Castiglione, B. (1561/1948) *The Book of the Courtier*, reprint, London: J.M. Dent and Sons.

Centers for Disease Control and Prevention (2005) *Diseases and Conditions*, retrieved 30 November 2005, from http://www.cdc.gov/node.do/id/0900f3ec8000e035

Channa Perera S.D. and Pollanen M.S. (2007) 'Sudden death due to sickle cell crisis during law enforcement restraint', *Journal of Forensic and Legal Medicine*, 14: 297–300.

Christie, W.F. (1927) *Surplus Fat and How to Reduce it*, London: Heinemann/Medical Books.

Conrad, P. (2005) 'The shifting engines of medicalization', *Journal of Health and Social Behaviour*, 46: 3–14.

Copeland, R.S. (1922) *Over Weight? Guard Your Health*, New York: Cosmopolitan.

Courtney, M. (ed.) (2005) *Evidence for Nursing Practice*, Sydney: Churchill Livingstone.

Crandall, C. (1994) 'Prejudice against fat people: ideology and self-interest', *Journal of Personality and Social Psychology*, 66: 882–94.

Croskerry, P. (2002) 'Achieving quality in clinical decision making: cognitive strategies and detection of bias', *Academic Emergency Medicine*, 9: 1184–205.

Dicenso, A., Guyatt, G. and Ciliska, D. (2005) *Evidence-based Nursing,* St Louis, MO: Elsevier Mosby.

Dixon, J. and Banwell, C. (2004) 'Re-embedding trust: unravelling the construction of modern diets', *Critical Public Health,* 14: 117–31.

Eisenberg, L. and Kleinman, A. (1980) 'Clinical Social Science', in L. Eisenberg and A. Kleinman (eds) *The Relevance of Social Science for Medicine,* Dordrecht, ND: D. Reidel Publishing Company.

Foucault, M. (1963) *Naissance de la Clinique,* Paris: Presses Universitaires de France.

General Mills (2008) *BMI Calculator,* retrieved 9 February 2008, from http://www.generalmills.com/corporate/health_wellness/bmi_calculator. aspx?section=fitnut&sub=bmi

Gevitz, N. (2000) '"The devil hath laughed at the physicians": Witchcraft and medical practice in seventeenth-century New England', *Journal of the History of Medicine,* 55: 5–36.

Guggenheim, K.Y. (1995) 'Chlorosis: the rise and disappearance of a nutritional disease,' *The Journal of Nutrition,* 125: 1822–5.

Hamilton, J., Campos, R. and Creed, F. (1996) 'Anxiety, depression and management of medically unexplained symptoms in medical clinics', *Journal of the Royal College of Physicians London,* 30:18–20.

Haynes, R.B., Sackett, D.L., Taylor, D.W., Gibson, E.S. and Johnson, A.L. (1978) 'Increased absenteeism from work after detection and labeling of hypertensive patients', *New England Journal of Medicine,* 299: 741–744.

Hebl, M.R. and Xu, J. (2001) 'Weighing the care: physicians' reactions to the size of a patient', *International Journal of Obesity & Related Metabolic Disorders,* 25: 1246–52.

Herrick, S.S. (1889) 'Obesity', in A.H. Buck (ed.) *A Reference Handbook of the Medical Sciences,* Edinburgh: Pentland.

Hippocrates (1978) 'A Regimen for Health', in *Hippocratic Writings,* trans. C. and W.N. Mann, Harmondsworth: Penguin.

Holmes, D., Murray, S.J., Perron, A. and Rail, G. (2006) 'Deconstructing the evidence-based discourse in health sciences: truth, power and fascism', *International Journal of Evidence-based Health Care,* 4: 180–6.

Illich, I. (1976) *Limits to Medicine–Medical Nemesis: The Expropriation of Health.* Middlesex, GB: Penguin.

Jenny Craig (2008) *BMI Calculator: What's Your BMI score?,* retrieved 9 February 2008, from http://www.jennycraig.com/page/bmi.

Joint Committee on the Medico–Actuarial Mortality Investigation (1013) *Influence of Build on Mortality Among Men,* New York: Association of Life Insurance Medical Directors and Actuarial Society of America.

Jutel, A. (2001) 'Does size really matter? Weight and values in public health', *Perspectives in Biology and Medicine,* 44: 283–96.

———. (2006) 'The emergence of overweight as a disease category: measuring up normality', *Social Science and Medicine,* 63: 2268–76.

Jutel, A. and Buetow, S.A. (2007) 'A Picture of Health? Unmasking the role of appearance in health', *Perspectives in Biology and Medicine,* 50: 421–34.

Leray, J. (1931) *Embonpoint et Obésité: conceptions et thérapeutiques actuelles,* Paris: Massion et Cie.

Les Mills (2006) *World Health Organization Urges Activity,* retrieved 8 August 2006, from www.lesmills.co.nz.

McEntee, M. (2003) 'Health screenings: A tool for today's marketers', *Medical Marketing & Media,* 38: 52–9.

MacLaren, J.P. (1929) *Medical Insurance Examination: Modern Methods and Rating of Lives,* London: Bailliere, Tindall and Cox.

Mendelson, G. (2003) 'Homosexuality and psychiatric nosology', *Australia New Zealand Journal of Psychiatry*, 37: 678–83.

Morse, J.M. (2006) 'The politics of evidence', *Qualitative Health Research*, 16: 395–404.

Moynihan, R. and Henry, D. (2006) 'The fight against disease mongering: generating knowledge for action', *Public Library of Science Medicine*, 3(4): e191.

National Institutes of Health (1998) *Clinical Guidelines on the Identification, Evaluation, and Treatment of Overweight and Obesity in Adults*, Washington DC: US Department of Health and Human Services.

Oliver, J.E. (2006) 'The politics of pathology: how obesity became an epidemic disease', *Perspectives in Biology and Medicine*, 49: 611–29.

Pabst Brewing Company (1897) 'Pabst Malt Extract', *Godey's Magazine*.

Paquette M. (2003) 'Excited delirium: does it exist?', *Perspectives in Psychiatric Care*, 39: 93–4.

Quetelet, A. (1871) *Anthropométrie ou Mesure des Différentes Facultés de l'Homme*, Brussels: C. Muquardt.

Rolfe, G. (2005) 'The deconstructing angel: nursing, reflection and evidence-based practice', *Nursing Inquiry*, 12: 78–86.

Rony, H.R. (1940) *Obesity and Leanness*, Philadelphia: Lea & Febiger.

Rosenberg, C.E. (2002) 'The tyranny of diagnosis: specific entities and individual experience', *The Milbank Quarterly*, 80: 237–60.

Sackett, D.L., Straus, S.E., Richardson, W.S., Rosenberg, W. and Haynes, R.B. (2000) *Evidence-based Medicine: How to practice and teach EBM*, Edinburgh: Churchill Livingstone.

Schwartz, H. (1986) *Never Satisfied: A Cultural History of Diets, Fantasies and Fat*, New York: Anchor Books.

Schwinn Fitness (2006) *126/226 Exercise Bike Owner's Manual*, retrieved 26 December 2006, from http://download.dfxi.com/manuals/schwinn/SCH_126–226_OM_RevB_0906_web.pdf

Spitzack, C. (1990) *Confessing Excess: Women and the Politics of Body Reduction*, Albany, NY: State University of New York Press.

Stafford, B., La Puma, B. and Schiedermayer, D. (1989) 'One face of beauty, one picture of health: the hidden aesthetic of medical practice', *Journal of Medicine and Philosophy*, 14: 213–30.

Stearns, P. (1997) *Fat History: Bodies and Beauty in the Modern West*, New York: New York University Press.

Straus, S.E., Richardson, W.S., Glasziou, P. and Haynes, R.B. (2005) *Evidence-based Medicine*, Edinburgh: Elsevier Churchill Livingstone.

The Lancet (1897) 'The reliance personal weighing machine', *The Lancet*, 8 May: 1316.

Thomas, J. (1891) *A Complete Pronouncing Medical Dictionary*, London: Deacon.

Total Gym (2008) *How Fit Are You?*, retrieved 9 February 2008, from http://www.totalgymdirect.com/bmi.php

Zola, I.K. (1983) *Socio-Medical Inquiries: Recollections, Reflections, and Reconsiderations*, Philadelphia: Temple University Press.

———. (1986) 'Illness Behaviour: A Political Analysis', in McHugh, S. and Vallis, T.M. (eds) *Illness Behaviour: A Multi-Disciplinary Model*, New York: Plenum Press.

6 Marked as 'Pathological'

'Fat' Bodies as Virtual Confessors

Samantha Murray

Food, dieting, exercise, and movement provide meanings, values, norms, and ideals that the subject actively ingests, incorporating social categories into the physiological interior. Bodies speak, without necessarily talking, because they become coded with and as signs. They speak social codes. They become intextuated, narrativized; simultaneously, social codes, laws, norms, and ideals become incarnated.

(Grosz 1995: 35)

In *Space, Time & Perversion* Elizabeth Grosz (1995) suggests that as subjects, we come to attach certain social and cultural codings to the aesthetic appearance of all bodies (including the 'obese' subject). In other words, it is in and through processes of socialisation that we are subjected to a *biopedagogy* of normative bodily aesthetics: that is, the ways in which we maintain our bodies, and co-extensively, the ways in which our bodies (and the bodies of others) appear in the world come to discursively 'mean' particular things to us. Given this, we acquire the means to 'read' and understand certain bodies as 'confessing' supposed 'truths' about one's being. Grosz (1995: 34–5) goes on to focus her critical attention on the understanding of all bodies as 'virtual confessors', and asserts that '[t]he body becomes a text, a system of signs to be deciphered, read, and read into. While social law is incarnate, "corporealized", correlatively, bodies are textualized, "read" by others as *expressive* of a subject's psychic interior'.

Visible bodily markers (such as fat flesh) are read in ways that position subjects on either the 'acceptable' or 'unacceptable' side of the normal/pathological binary equation that signify subjects as either adhering to the requirements of 'healthy' ethical living, or as engaging in 'unhealthy' behaviours that position one as a moral and aesthetic failure. Following on from this argument, it is my task in this chapter to demonstrate that the fundamental intercorporeality of social space exhibits the visible bodily markers that have been discursively produced as representing/constructing normativity or pathology. In unpacking this notion, I specifically look at the act of 'confession', particularly in the space of the clinic between doctor and 'fat' patient. The fat body is always already *'seen'*, and the privilege of *visibility* is its purported correlative to *knowledge*. Here, I stage a challenge to medical discourses/narratives that constitute 'obesity' as a disease, and, particularly, to elucidate the power and authority of the medical voice in making 'fat' bodies intelligible as pathological and immoral, not simply to doctors, but to the 'fat' individual. Thus, I look specifically at the constructions of individual responsibility that are evident in medical narratives and discourses about 'obesity', and the effects of (what I argue) is the forced 'confession' of a deficient self residing in a 'fat' body.

As Grosz demonstrates, bodies are considered, in our culture at least, to confess a 'truth', and while there may not be a singular ideal, there are certainly dominant ones. In reading the ways in which bodies 'speak' as Grosz posits, we rely on (and are compelled by) a liberal humanist (and necessarily, individualistic) logic that ignores the fundamental intercorporeality of our being-in-the-world, to instead insist that bodies are an external expression of an *inner self*: hence, visible bodily markers of difference must signal more fundamental aberrations of the 'self'. Grosz notes that in the individualist assumptions that continue to govern public notions of self-transformation and self-authorship, what is neglected is 'the problem of other minds' (Grosz 1994: 12) that always already code bodies and give them meaning. The practice of reading the bodies of others is not something that is deployed only at the level of the individual reading the body of another, but is part of a larger system of exchange whereby the reading of one's body *inscribes* that body with particular meanings, and (re)produces the psychic world of the subject being 'read'. As part of the continuing dominance of humanist logic in medical narratives and public health discourse, the body stands as an *exhibition* of a subject's biopedagogy and one's moral investment in 'health/normality'—a 'healthy' body then is perceived to reveal the 'healthy' truth of the interior life-world of the subject. While medicine relies on a separation of mind and body, the two inevitably inform and construct each other as *part* of the humanist logic it is founded on.

MORAL MEDICINE: CONSTITUTING ETHICAL BODIES

In the esteemed *Medical Journal of Australia*, physician John Burry (1999) published a paper entitled, 'Obesity and Virtue: Is Staying Lean a Matter of Ethics?'. Burry's core argument is that in spite of medical evidence to suggest 'obesity' is a genetic inheritance, maintaining a 'healthy' weight is the responsibility of every individual, and is indeed a matter of ethics. In other words, Burry constructs weight control as what Christine Halse (see Chapter 4 in this collection) describes as a 'virtue discourse'. Burry (1999: 2–3) argues:

> Control of weight, no matter that some have a genetically determined potential to acquire and retain more weight in comparison with others,

remains a matter of self-control and personal responsibility . . . This responsibility is related to personal health and the health of offspring, and to the health costs and the healthy functioning of the general community . . . In a liberal society, fulfilling this responsibility must be a matter of voluntary behaviour, as "personal autonomy, the right to choose one's own way of life for oneself, is the supreme value" . . . Self-control of one's weight might be described as a form of bioethics.

Burry's thesis exposes not only the humanist/individualist logic of modern medical practice, it demonstrates the inextricability of morality and the 'proper' bodily aesthetics of 'healthy' bodies. Given the oft-proclaimed 'objectivity' of medicine, it is telling that the very ways in which we separate 'pathological' bodies from 'normal' bodies is just as much about upholding morality as it is about 'health'. What is also revealed is the tacit assumption that 'obese' subjects are 'immoral' subjects. For Burry, their 'fatness' is evidence of their neglect of a correct 'ethics of the body': they are explicit moral and ethical failures that are positioned as unethical and unwilling to assume a 'proper' responsibility for their health and, as Halse suggests, the health of the nation. Within this, I would argue, is Burry's contempt for 'fat' patients who have neglected a 'moral' ethics of bodily maintenance, veiled by a medical concern for the health problem of 'obesity'. The fat body, for Burry, is a 'virtual confessor' that is, fat flesh always already confesses a pathology, by virtue of its very visible difference. However, what appears to be most maddening for Burry is the seeming *denial* of this virtual confession pathology by a fat subject who will not conform to his 'virtuous mean'. I will discuss this notion in greater detail shortly.

While Burry (1999: 3) contends that 'obesity' has been shown to occur more often in poorer socio-economic areas, and says that '[e]xercising personal responsibility involves a minimum social, economic, political and educational understanding', he goes on to insist, 'I do not wish to deny that there are social elements to the problem, but we need a motivating framework for those who have practical autonomy yet cannot control their weight' (Burry 1999: 3). Included in his argument is the following recommendation: 'Politicians, clergy, police and moral philosophers must lead the way in physical fitness if we are to expect to reap the benefits of a lean society' (Burry 1999: 3).

Burry's call to action echoes the recommendations of public health directives about obesity across the Western world,[1] in mobilising people 'of influence' to endorse the edicts of the medical authorities, and act as moral superiors. What exactly *are* the benefits of a 'lean' society? And more specifically, exactly *who* is benefited? Is Burry encouraging a kind of 'moral cleansing' in asking public figures to preach through their bodies an aesthetic of 'slenderness' that equates to health?

In this article Burry is tacitly attaching a moral value to 'thinness' as the status quo for a proper sense of nationhood and citizenship. This is evident in the conclusion to the article where Burry (1999: 3) summons a discourse of 'virtue', stating '[l]et us propose a BMI of 22 to 25 as "virtuous mean" to which we should all aspire'. Burry suggests that by engaging in processes deemed to be indicative of a moral commitment (that is, weight loss) you may be restored to an ethical citizen. In a secular Western world, bodily maintenance has become the most visible signifier of morality and one's adherence to the dictates of an ethical lifestyle. This notion is elaborated by Peter Stearns (1997: 247), who writes:

> Dieting is fascinating beyond its role as a daily constraint because of what it may say about other moral uncertainties in modern life, because of its redefinition and standardization of physical beauty, and because of its symbolic testimony to good character and personal discipline.

Taking into account Burry's (1999) argument, what is evident is the degree to which disciplinary medicine relies on the presence of the spectre of morality as a necessary effect of control and regulation to preserve in individuals the autonomous belief in one's own ability to know oneself, to master one's body and self-mastery. Burry's commitment to numerical values as a 'virtuous mean' by which to measure oneself demonstrates the necessary intermingling of medical science and moral values attached to quantification of certain bodies in marking normativity. Established by medical authority, and traded as a kind of currency between members of lay society are these numbers: kilograms, Body Mass Indexes (BMI), body fat ratios. These numerical values carry moral import as tools to fabricate normative bodies as aspirational ideals that are nonetheless fundamentally immaterial. Annemarie Jutel asserts in 'Does Size Really Matter? Weight and Values in Public Health' that there is an 'over-reliance on weight as an indicator of health' (Jutel 2001: 1), and that these numerical quantifications of bodies have serious implications for medical attitudes towards 'obese' subjects. This can be noted in the way in which 'doctors are less likely to investigate lifestyle choices or even to provide health advice to slender patients than they are to heavy ones' (Jutel, 2001: 1). Jutel (2001: 3) goes on to claim that:

> Mirroring early beliefs that physical imperfections reflect inner shortcomings, contemporary physicians unconsciously use visual and perceptual judgements in their evaluation of health, drawing their patients into an aesthetic of normality. As a result, geometrical concepts, numbers, and proportions support definitions of health. "Capturing" normality in a formula, or proportion, such as a height–weight chart, reflects moral and aesthetics judgements about how one ought to look. These views play an important role in the management of the "problem" of overweight. In Western society, values of homogeneity and visual aesthetics guide our judgements of what is good and healthy, and imprint themselves firmly on our approach to weight management.

Jutel notes the authority of these quantification formulas in medicine, but also in their ready deployment outside the clinic between lay subjects. The equalising function of a number, or a 'virtuous mean' as Burry (1999) describes it, to which we should all subscribe, is a powerful means of control that taps into a fundamental desire to achieve normative status, and to understand oneself as occupying the privileged position of 'health' in the health/pathology binary equation. Nikolas Rose highlights the powerful effects of mobilising the authority of medicine in weight loss directives about bodily maintenance and self-regulation. He writes:

> The infusion of medical values into ethical judgements can be located in relation to the successive ways in which humans have been urged to engage in practices of self-formation, to master themselves, improve themselves and regulate themselves in the name of certain problems and through the use of certain techniques.
>
> (Rose 1994: 69)

'FAT' BODIES AS VIRTUAL CONFESSORS

Without our volition or control, then, the body *always already confesses*. In *The History of Sexuality: Volume One*, Michel Foucault (1978) asserts that since the middle ages, the West has made increasing use of the rite of confession in the production of truth. Whether in church, the clinic, or on the street, the act of 'confession' has become key to the operation of knowledge/power, and demonstrates the ways in which we have embodied the biopedagogy of 'proper' bodies. Foucault (1978: 63) asserts the dispersed nature of the disciplinary power associated with the confessional, stating '[the confession] gradually lost its ritualistic and exclusive localization; it spread; it has been employed in a whole series of relationships: children and parents, students and educators, patients and psychiatrists, delinquents and experts'. Foucault notes that where we originally relied on the testimonies of others to illustrate one's character, we now mobilize confession in pronouncing the truth of ourselves. Such is the power of the confession in the West as a tool in the production of 'truth' that it has pervaded every aspect of our contemporary lives: in personal relationships, juridical matters, and medical consultation. What most interests Foucault about confession is that it plays a central role in *individualisation*, in the systems of identity and difference, systems of categorisation, and the systems of reward and punishment that are attached to these categories that pivot around the binary of normalcy/deviance. He claims:

> One confesses—or is forced to confess. When it is not spontaneous or dictated by some internal imperative, the confession is wrung from a

person by violence or threat, it is driven from its hiding place in the soul or extracted from the body.

(Foucault 1978: 59)

Foucault's theory of confession has interesting implications for the 'obese' body of medical discourse. All bodies are always already visible: with regard to the 'obese' body, its pathology is inscribed onto its 'fat' flesh through the 'expert' medical interpretation of its simultaneous characterisation as 'diseased', and as a body unwilling to recognize its disease. The incitement to confess (that takes place not only in the clinic, but in a myriad of social spaces) is based on a demand for the 'obese' subject's *own recognition* of pathology, of an *ownership* of a body of transgressions. The confessee has read and 'knows' the body of the 'obese' confessor as a body of disease and excess, in and through historically and culturally specific discourses that have become sedimented in our very being at an almost pre-conscious level, and are mobilized in the practice of reading bodies without conscious or deliberate effort. In this way, it would seem the confession of the 'fat' body is already foretold. Let me elucidate this. There seems to be an implicit silencing in the extraction of a confession from the 'fat' body. The irony is that as the bodily markers of the 'fat' body are read, they provide 'access to a subjectivity' (Alcoff 2001: 268). In this way, the 'obese' subject is immediately 'known': the 'fat' flesh of one's body has already silently performed a confession. This confession is one of necessary pathology, indulgence and excess, and before the 'fat' subject even speaks, this confession is produced as a truth. The fat body always already virtually confesses, and thus an interior 'truth' is supposedly assigned to the fat subject, for them to then admit and confirm. Foucault (1978: 60) asserts:

> The obligation to confess . . . is so deeply ingrained in us, that we no longer perceive it as the effect of a power that constrains us; on the contrary, it seems to us that truth, lodged in our most secret nature "demands" only to surface . . . Confession frees—but power reduces one to silence . . . production [of truth] is thoroughly imbued with relations of power.

Foucault (1978) points out that a confession always requires a subject to have someone to confess to—and to thus exercise on the confessing subject the power of exoneration, redemption, judgement, or punishment. The ritual of the confession involves power relations that act upon the body of the confessing subject, whereby an essential 'truth' has been revealed and the body–subject must be policed, and (self) regulated. In Foucault's portrait of confession, the function of power, specific to the 'obese' woman, is the confirmation of the knowledges that govern the relationship between the confessor and the confessee: as Foucault (1978: 59) says, 'in between the words, a truth [emerges] which the very form of the confession holds out like a shimmering mirage'. A confession is not a self-realisation or a revelation to the one who hears the confession; rather it is structured as a moment of confirmation of the tacit knowledges that form the perceptual background to the power relations operating between the confessor and the confessee. The confessee is positioned as *already knowing* the 'truth', but wants to *confirm* the confessor is also aware of the truth of their own body. Such is the function of the disciplinary power of norms and pathologies, well beyond the walls of the clinic. As Foucault (1978: 61–2) suggests:

> The confession is a ritual of discourse in which the speaking subject is also the subject of the statement; it is also a ritual that unfolds within a power relationship, for one does not confess without the presence (or virtual presence) of a partner who is not simply the interlocutor but the authority who requires the confession, prescribes it and appreciates it, and intervenes in order to judge, punish, forgive, console, and reconcile; a ritual in which the truth is corroborated by the obstacles and resistances it has had to surmount in order to be formulated.

Having lived as a fat woman, on several occasions I have consulted with doctors about various maladies I was suffering from, which I was invariably told were a direct result of what they perceived as my 'fatness'. Via the 'clinical gaze' of the doctor, my fat body was always already pathological by virtue of its hypervisibility. Of course, the clinical examination of my body would also involve the doctor deploying various technological apparatuses aimed at enhancing their perception (blood pressure monitors, stethoscopes, x-rays, ultrasounds and so on) in order to confirm the doctor's diagnosis of my fat body as pathological, with the usual range of co-morbidities such as diabetes, heart disease, hypertension and joint problems. Maddeningly, in the wake of these investigations, my doctors were forced to conclude (albeit somewhat disappointedly) that my blood pressure was in fact 'normal', my lung capacity was 'good', and my internal organs were in working order. Nevertheless, under the medical gaze, the eminent visibility of my 'diseased', 'obese' body functioned as a signifier of *pathology*, my 'bodily being' was perceived by those concerned, as a negative, 'problematic' mode of embodiment. I was repeatedly advised to lose weight as a matter of urgency, despite my otherwise apparently good 'health'.

While the doctors I consulted immediately perceived me as 'fat', in order for me to accept (even in part) the pathological label of 'obesity', what was required was a confession of my own pathology. As Foucault claims, this exchange is far from neutral, but is only legitimized and validated if the confessee is positioned as a subject of authority who holds the power to forgive, correct, alter or transform the newly purged confessor. The diagnostic procedure, then, can be said to be marked by the *confessional*. However, the confession of the patient is not offered as an unadulterated 'truth'. The confession must be filtered, and interpreted by the authority embodied by the *one confessed to*. Foucault (1978: 66) demonstrates this here:

> If one had to confess, this was not merely because the person to whom one confessed had the power to forgive, console, and direct, but because the work of producing the truth was obliged to pass through this relationship if it was to be scientifically validated. The truth did not reside solely in the subject who, by confessing would reveal it wholly formed. It was constituted in two stages: present but incomplete, blind to itself, in the one who spoke, it could only reach completion in the one who assimilated and recorded it.

The diagnosis handed from the doctor to the patient undergoes a tacit negotiation before this is accepted. What is most interesting here is the marking of the confessional again by a humanist logic. The patient/child/prisoner is invited into a space that is simultaneously marked by apparent autonomy, where the confessor is given the 'opportunity' to reveal a truth of themselves, while at the same time, a disciplinary power functions to hear this confession, interpret it, and to produce a 'truth' *for* the confessor. This negotiation is effected through the power relations present in the hearing of a confession of pathology from the patient. This moment of confession verifies the patient's pathology, and inscribes the pathology onto the patient as a 'truth'. As Margrit Shildrick (1997: 48) explains:

> In this, the sciences of man, of which Foucault characterizes modern medicine as the first example . . . are exemplary in that they constitute the individual in terms of a series of norms, while at the same time inviting the subject to produce truths about herself.

Similarly, in *Corporeal Generosity*, Rosalyn Diprose (2002) locates the doctor's consulting rooms and the clinical encounter that takes place within these walls as a site of confession. Diprose speaks of sexuality in her discussion, but I would suggest that a similar confessional trajectory occurs in the clinical encounter with a 'fat' patient. Diprose (2002: 109–10) suggests:

> In this medical examination we are not simply confessing to an already constituted sexuality and unburdening ourselves of a truth that seems to infect us. Rather . . . we are constituting ourselves as subjects of sexuality in the presence of someone with the authority to make of us what she will.

By this, Diprose means that in the moment of confessing one's supposed 'pathology' one *(re)makes* oneself, *(re)producing* oneself as a subject of this pathology and what this pathology *means* culturally, in a (clinical) space where one is most vulnerable, where one is seeking help and reassurance.

Diprose (2002:110) says that '[t]he clinic, like the confessional in general, incites not just the desire to speak but desire itself. It is a place where pleasures and pains are articulated, formed, and transformed; where a self is dissolved, dissembled, and assembled'. Diprose (2002: 111–12) uses a story in her discussion that I would like to recount in part here:

> Claudia enters a clinic seeking a prescription for her asthma medication. She knows what she needs, and this is all she wants. The doctor, a woman around Claudia's age and unfamiliar with her case, asks the usual two or three questions about Claudia's medical history before happily meeting her request. But as she is writing the prescription, the doctor asks if there is anything else that Claudia would like. Even though Claudia replies "no" several times, the doctor persists: did Claudia realize, for instance, that a simple course of hormone therapy could eliminate her problem of facial hair. Claudia is . . . mortified by this question.

Diprose (2002: 114) comments that in light of stories like Claudia's '[i]t is clear . . . that . . . the clinician is an agency of domination, a deputy of medical discourse and the conventions it may harbour'. Claudia's body is offered up in the clinical space, and as it is read within the rubrics of dominant discourses about feminine beauty (to which the clinician cannot be immune), Claudia's body confesses without her uttering a word, just as the 'fat' body appears as pathological before the patient has even spoken to complain about a possible unrelated malaise.

Similarly, in Marcia Millman's (1980) landmark book *Such a Pretty Face: Being Fat in America*, the author talks about the indignities of the 'fat' woman's experience of going to the doctor. It has been thought that the percentage of obese women with life-threatening diseases is often higher than women of a normal weight, because they are unwilling to seek medical help for fear of derision and humiliation. This is poignantly evident in the following story recounted to Millman:

> I've had a lot of bad experiences with . . . doctors in general. A fat person hates to go to the doctor. Even if you go to the doctor because of a cold, the doctor will say "lose 50 pounds" as if that will take care of the cold . . . I had a cold, walked into [the doctor's] office and he looked at me and said, "I'm not going to treat you unless you lose some weight". I said, "I just want some cough medicine so I won't cough myself to death". He said, "Okay. I'll give you some cough medicine, but if you don't lose 20 pounds in two weeks, don't come back".
>
> (Millman 1980: 18)

In both of the examples offered above, the clinician appears to attempt to *wrest* a confession of pathology from the patient, as though the primary complaint of a cold that had brought the patient to the doctor's office in the first place was some sort of elaborate ruse to enter the space of confession, to unburden oneself of one's pathology. Whether the confessional operates within or outside of the church, the effect is the same. Attached to the 'truth' produced for the confessor is a moral value that is marked by the presence of pathology. The 'normative', 'healthy' body (which is most often represented in public health discourse as a 'thin' body) speaks to its society of an adherence to tenets of purity and maintenance of the body through self-control and managed desires. However, this venerated body is a fundamentally immaterial one. By this, I mean to suggest that this 'normative' body is nowhere to be found a reality. Despite its ideal status, and its function as a 'phantasy', its aspirational power lies in the privilege it affords. Given this 'normative slender' body's immateriality, all bodies fail as projects, albeit to varying degrees and with different cultural values attached to their respective failings. In discussing the particularity of the cultural values attached to the perceived 'failing' of the 'fat' woman's body, Spitzack (1990: 31) suggests, '[a]s one who is diseased physically and morally, the obese woman is obliged culturally to "admit" to her sins and abnormalities'. This obligation to confess is thrown into higher relief given the permeation of medical attitudes about 'obesity' beyond the walls of the clinic and into a popular consciousness. Thomas Osborne (1998: 270) discusses the function and implications of naturalising norms beyond the clinic:

> For, when the principle is taken up within other disciplines, it supports the positivist contention that the normal can be known and laid down as law, prior to the pathological. In short, we get a general obsession not with a given human nature but with normality as such. Such is another consequence of a medical ideology: something which may be unremarkable in narrowly medical terms, but which has powers, so to speak, beyond itself, as a principle of transferability.

By *transferability*, Osborne asserts that medicine has extended beyond itself, and that 'normalisation' and 'pathologisation' have become social phenomena. 'In short, the very "power" of medicine is dependent upon its status as ideology in this particular sense; where norms stray beyond themselves' (Osborne 1998: 271). Indeed, the norm/pathology binary has constructed us as subjects, has enabled our readings of our own bodies and the bodies of others, and requires 'othered' fat bodies to confess their difference: to confess their pathology, their moral failure, and their aesthetic affront. What I have attempted to demonstrate here is the complex and fraught interrelationships between medical and popular discourse, normative bodily aesthetics, and morality. Moreover, what I have shown is the ways is which these interrelationships inform and support each other, and the implications they have for the lived embodiment of those marked and positioned as unethical, immoral and pathological.

CONCLUSIONS

Terry and Urla (1995: 1) argue that medical discourse is always already shot through with moral imaginings of the 'proper' body:

> With early roots in Aristotelian comparative studies, the idea that moral character is rooted in the body has structured a wide variety of modern medical and scientific studies, and shapes the current conditions under which popular fictions circulate about the bodies of all kinds of people who are deemed to be in some way behaviourally aberrant or socially disruptive.

By drawing on Terry and Urla's claims about the permeation of medical discourses in popular culture and everyday intersubjective encounters, and in order to conclude my discussion, I would like to mention briefly an Australian public health campaign against 'obesity'. This initiative, titled *I Decide*, was launched by Abbott Australasia (2002a), the pharmaceutical company responsible for one of the more recent weight loss drugs, Xenical (orlistat). The campaign features an extensive television commercial series, which consists of a number of both male and female 'clinically obese' participants, promising the camera such things as 'I will not eat that slice of cake', 'I will exercise more', 'I will listen to my doctor', which is followed up with the tagline of the campaign 'I Decide'. Campaign posters are visible in many pharmacies and doctor's offices, with images of the smiling actors from the television commercials, with the words 'I Decide' running under their faces. What is not immediately evident to the general public about this campaign is that it is in fact a marketing campaign for a weight loss drug that has recently has its status changed by national medical authorities so that it can now be purchased over-the-counter without a doctor's prescription. The *I Decide* campaign launched a website (http://www.idecide.com.au) that provides readers with a number of different 'tools' and resources for their weight loss, such as BMI calculators, tips for finding a doctor to assist you, exercise and eating plans and suggestions such as keeping a 'food diary' in order to track daily exactly what foods you consume. The website homepage features a real-time clock ticking down the seconds, with the question in bold lettering underneath: 'Is this the moment you decide to talk to your doctor about your weight?'. Below this is the caption: 'Weight loss begins from within' (Abbott Australasia 2006a). In the section entitled 'Talking With Your Doctor', the following advice is given:

> Losing weight needs a commitment from you. Explain you have taken a real decision to lose weight and that you are conscious about sensible eating and the importance of exercise—but you would also like to know more about treatments your doctor can offer and what other assistance they can give.
>
> (Abbott Australasia 2002b)

The *I Decide* campaign is reliant upon the *admission* and *acknowledgement* of the 'obese' subject of one's pathology and deficiency, a gesture that is, in itself, constitutive: in short, 'I Decide' could be rebranded to read 'I Confess'. The campaign operates under the disguise of permitting subjects to *choose*: '*I decide*', it is up to me, *I* make the choice about *my* health and *my* body. What the *I Decide* program requires from its participants is a confession, where the images of the actors used in the promotional posters and banners, despite hesitant and/or satisfied smiles, appear as a kind of mugshot, zeroing in on the 'obese' subject's face, waiting for a confession. The '*decision*' to lose weight is an expected correlative to the '*confession*' of one's 'fat' pathology.

Moreover, the campaign is reliant on the visibility of fat flesh, of the way we code fatness as aberrant, both aesthetically and clinically. It demands that the fat faces of the subjects featured in the campaign posters be read by us, to be positioned by us as pathological, and as confessing to their bodily neglect. While operating under the rubric of a medically necessary lifestyle change, the obese subjects in the *I Decide* campaign command us to read their bodily difference, and to approve their decision/confession not simply because of a health danger, but in light of the aesthetic affront their fatness poses. This public health campaign is disciplinary/surveillance medicine in action: 'obese' Australians are asked to recognize themselves in the faces of the 'fat' actors featured in the posters, and to bear witness to their own pathology. One's 'decision', one's imputed autonomy belies a more fundamental mobilisation of the health/pathology binary, whereby health is presented in a clearly understood model/bodily aesthetic, where 'obese' subjects are expected (ironically) to confess their bodily transgression, and must then 'decide', choose to normalize themselves. Juxtaposed with the conviction of a personal autonomy and choice in one's relation to one's body, the act of 'confession' requires the other to normalize oneself, and to be 'healthy'.

NOTES

1. See, for example, the World Health Organisation's action plan (2000) that addresses the 'global obesity epidemic': *Obesity: preventing and managing the global epidemic*, Geneva: World Health Organisation. See also an Australian strategic plan for obesity treatment written by the National Health and Medical Research Council (NHMRC) (1997) *Acting on Australia's Weight: summary report*, Canberra: Australian Government Publishing Service.

REFERENCES

Abbott Australasia (2006a) *I Decide*, retrieved 21 March 2006, from http://www.idecide.com.au

Abbott Australasia (2006b) *Talking with your doctor*, retrieved 21 March 2006, from http://www.idecide.com.au/index.php?id=10

Alcoff, L.M. (2001) 'Towards a Phenomenology of Racial Embodiment', in R. Bernasconi (ed.) *Race*, Malden, MA: Blackwell Publishers.

Burry, J.N. (1999) 'Obesity and virtue: is staying lean a matter of ethics?', *The Medical Journal of Australia*, 171: 609–10.

Diprose, R. (2002) *Corporeal Generosity: On Giving With Nietzsche, Merleau-Ponty, and Levinas*, Albany, NY: State University of New York Press.

Foucault, M. (1978) *The History of Sexuality Volume 1: AnIntroduction*, trans. R. Hurley, London: Penguin Books.

Grosz, E. (1994) *Volatile Bodies: Toward a Corporeal Feminism*, St Leonards, Sydney: Allen & Unwin.

———. (1995) *Space, Time & Perversion: The Politics of Bodies*, St Leonards, Sydney: Allen & Unwin.

Jutel, A. (2001) 'Does size really matter? Weight and values in public health'. *Perspectives in Biology and Medicine*, 44(2): 283–96.

Millman, M. (1980) *Such a Pretty Face: Being Fat in America*, New York and London: W.W. Norton & Company.

National Health and Medical Research Council (NHMRC) (1997) *Acting on Australia's Weight: Summary Report*, Canberra: Australian Government Publishing Service.

Osborne, T. (1998) 'Medicine and ideology', *Economy and Society*, 27(2 & 3): 259–73.

Rose, N. (1994) 'Medicine, History and the Present', in C. Jones and R. Porter (eds) *Reassessing Foucault: Power, Medicine and the Body*, New York; London: Routledge.

Shildrick, M. (1997) *Leaky Bodies and Boundaries: Feminism, Postmodernism and (Bio)Ethics*, New York and London: Routledge.

Spitzack, C. (1990) *Confessing Excess: Women and the Politics of Body Reduction*, Albany, NY: State University of New York Press.

Stearns, P. (1997) *Fat History: Bodies and Beauty in the Modern West*, New York: New York University Press.

Terry, J. and Urla, J. (1995) 'Introduction: Mapping Embodied Deviance', in J. Terry and J. Urla (eds) *Deviant Bodies: Critical Perspectives on Difference in Science and Popular Culture*, Bloomington: Indiana University Press.

World Health Organisation (2000) Obesity: Preventing and Managing the Global Epidemic, Geneva: World Health Organisation.

Part II

Governing Young People

Schools, Families and the 'Obesity Epidemic'

7 An Impossible Task?

Preventing Disordered Eating in the Context of the Current Obesity Panic

Natalie Beausoleil

INTRODUCTION

Currently, in Canada and elsewhere in the West, policy makers address issues of health and wellness of the population mostly through campaigns focused on individual lifestyles, namely 'healthy eating' and 'active living'. This chapter takes a critical stance with regards to this particular health promotion framework and argues that campaigns focused on individuals' lifestyles in fact contribute to increased disordered eating and growing body anxieties among the general population.

I write as a feminist researcher and a volunteer activist in the field of body image, body equity and the prevention of disordered eating. Following the crucial works of critical scholars Campos (2004), and Gard and Wright (2005), I argue that health professionals have wrongly conflated thinness with good health, on the one hand, and obesity/fatness and ill-health, on the other. Based on dubious health claims, obesity scientists have created a panic that unfortunately fosters further ill-health among the population (Campos 2004; Gard and Wright 2005). Dominant discourses of the 'healthy body' have paradoxically become instrumental in contributing to disordered eating, fat hatred and generalized destructive practices and obsessive anxieties about the body. The current obsession with individual health practices in the West may indeed prove to be very unhealthy.

The first section of this chapter describes some of the challenges and strategies activists and researchers promoting body equity face in the midst of contradictory, confusing and destructive messages conveyed in health promotion programs and policies in Canada. More specifically I critically reflect on my experience with the Body Image Network (BIN), a St John's-based non-profit organization composed of health professionals and volunteers who attempt to prevent disordered eating and promote a positive body image for people of all shapes and sizes in Newfoundland and Labrador. I discuss how difficult it is for BIN to advocate social change and go against very powerful regulatory discourses of 'health' and the 'healthy body' embedded in current health policies and school initiatives.

The second section of the chapter reports on the results of a study conducted among youth in St John's, Newfoundland, and Fredericton, New Brunswick, about their perceptions and practices of health and fitness. While the youth we talked with adopted the basic tenets of the dominant discourses of health, their narratives also show that young people's bodies are not completely regulated by the current socially prescribed health imperative. I conclude this chapter with my thoughts as a feminist researcher advocating for social change, a witness to powerful regulatory discourses and subtle instances of critical consciousness. In these spaces and moments when bodies are not completely disciplined, there is a seed of hope for a healthier society and collective empowerment of diverse bodies.

THEORETICAL AND METHODOLOGICAL CONSIDERATIONS

This chapter offers a feminist poststructuralist analysis of the relation between health promotion and the dominant discourses of health, weight, disordered eating and the body in contemporary western society. A poststructuralist framework is useful to understand how specific social relations, language and institutional practices constitute the domains of education and health that, in turn, affect how individuals will construct their sense of embodied self and identity (Rice 2007; Wright 2004). Poststructuralist discourse analysis fosters a critical examination of the socially constructed and historically located phenomena of health and the body. Discourses of the healthy body are particularly important in contemporary western society as a site of social control (Turner 1995 and 1996). In the contexts of the corporatization of health and the overall health panic in the west, individuals are required to be 'good citizens' by accepting the doctrine of, and acting upon, individual responsibility for health (Rail and Beausoleil 2003).

This chapter addresses social relations and the cultural meanings of body and health not only in dominant (or hegemonic) discourses but also in how people experience and embody cultural messages about health and self. This chapter is grounded in feminist theories of embodiment though I do not attempt here to review the literature in the field as this would go well beyond the scope of this chapter. The first section of the chapter discusses health promotion and the prevention of disordered eating from my perspective as co-founder and co-chair of the Body Image Network (BIN), a non-profit organization which aims to promote positive body image for all and prevent unhealthy and disordered eating in Newfoundland and Labrador.

The second section of the chapter is based on a broad project on youth's discursive constructions of health and fitness (Rail, Beausoleil, MacNeill, Burrows & Wright 2003).[1] This study investigates how youth take up dominant messages and construct their own notions of health and fitness. This research was also conducted in Ottawa and Toronto areas (see Rail chapter). In this chapter I will focus solely on the data collected in St John's,

Newfoundland and in Fredericton, New Brunswick. Between July 2004 and March 2005, we conducted altogether 14 semi-directed focus groups for a total of 76 participants (54 girls and 22 boys). Their ages ranged between 12 and 16 years and they came from a mix of working- and middle-classes, various ethnic groups and with diverse levels of physical activity. We recruited our participants via community organizations working with youth. A copy of the research proposal was granted ethical clearance from Memorial University's Human Investigation Committee (HIC).

The focus groups covered broad questions on how the participants define health, how they experience health and fitness in their own lives and in relations to others, and where they get their ideas about health. We also asked the participants to do individual drawings of a 'healthy' youth and a 'fit' youth and write comments on these drawings. For the purpose of this chapter I use only the data coming from our focus groups (all names used are pseudonyms). Based on a thematic analysis of the young people's narratives, I examine the ways in which cultural texts work to construct particular regimes of truth about health and fitness, and the ways in which the young people's meanings about health and fitness have been constructed in specific social and cultural circumstances. I therefore link the analysis of young people's talk to the larger social discourses and practices that shape how young people think about health and fitness.

HEALTH PROMOTION, THE BODY IMAGE NETWORK AND THE PREVENTION OF DISORDERED EATING

Obesity and the Prevention of Disordered Eating in Newfoundland and Labrador

Health officials have been particularly concerned with obesity in Newfoundland and Labrador since, according to Statistics Canada (2004), this province has the highest rate of obesity in the country. Official statistics also emphasize that children and youth in Newfoundland are not as active as other Canadian youth between the ages of 5–19 years old (CFLRI 2007). The Strategic Health Plan (Department of Health and Community Services 2002) and the Provincial Wellness Plan (Department of Health and Community Services 2006) for Newfoundland and Labrador aim to increase healthy behaviours and support services in the province. Alarmed by the 'high risk' factors of obesity and physical inactivity, the authors of both Plans call for initiatives and environments promoting healthier lifestyles (healthier diet and an increase in physical activity). In Newfoundland and Labrador, as in the rest of the country, policy makers have targeted youth and recommended that health curricula be revised and schools implement programs aimed at reducing obesity and encouraging healthy eating and physical activity among students. The initiative *Healthy Students, Healthy*

Schools, for instance, created jointly by the Department of Health and Community Services and the Department of Education, is intended to foster healthier eating and increased physical activity among students in Newfoundland and Labrador schools and larger community. This initiative is currently deployed in the province and has not been evaluated. However, researchers have assessed the impact of similar programs elsewhere. Some of these researchers note that the unintended effect of such programs may be for overweight children who are already at risk of low self-esteem to feel unacceptable (Walker Lowry, Sallinen and Janicke 2007). A recent study of the 'healthy eating, healthy weights' approach of the grades seven and eight Ontario health curriculum found that the focus on body monitoring and self-control in food choices for youth sent contradictory messages and increased weight anxieties for girls already struggling with body dissatisfaction (Larkin and Rice 2005). My own research among youth in this province shows that schools are crucial sites in the production of health and lifestyles discourses, an issue that I will explore in the next section.

While fighting obesity is very much on the minds of most policy makers, educators and health professionals in Newfoundland and Labrador, some have noticed body image distortions, disordered eating in general, and eating disorders in particular, in their interaction with youth in the province. As a result they have called on a specialized organization, the Body Image Network, to promote self-esteem and a positive body image for girls and boys, as well as for adults. Founded in 2000, the Body Image Network (BIN) consists of volunteers from a variety of disciplines and so includes sociologists, psychologists, dieticians, kinesiologists, nurses, epidemiologists, physicians, educators and students in various health related fields. Through education, awareness, research, advocacy and collaboration BIN encourages self-esteem and the respect of diverse bodies, eating well and being active.

The Body Image Network operated without funding until it received a Provincial Wellness grant in 2007 from the Department of Health and Community Services of the Government of Newfoundland and Labrador. Part of this grant involved developing a toolkit and updating presentations aimed at increasing self-esteem, body satisfaction and respect of diverse bodies, and broadening views towards healthy eating and physical activity practices. The goal of BIN is to help create a social environment that supports resilience to unrealistic expectations of the body. Over the years we (members of the Network) have given presentations to children, adolescents, and adults, health professionals, educators, the media and the general public. In an attempt to 'train the trainers' we plan to distribute our toolkit and presentations to various community leaders in the province such as teachers, group leaders (e.g. brownie and cub leaders), health professionals and coaches.

BIN's community involvement has recently fostered interesting alliances. BIN has been asked to formally take part in organizations addressing medically diagnosed eating disorders. The Eating Disorder working group (EDWG), a group of health professionals specializing in treatment of eating disorders within Eastern Health, asked BIN to join the group in order to cover prevention issues. The Eating Disorder Working Group had been operating for many years without including health promotion specialists. Moreover, the newly formed Eating Disorder Foundation of Newfoundland and Labrador (EDFNL), a province-wide advocacy group for people living with eating disorders and their families, has requested a representative of the BIN to sit on the Board of Directors. In recognizing that disordered eating is widespread beyond those who are currently diagnosed with an eating disorder, the Foundation and specifically members of the Board of Directors have looked for guidance from the BIN representative about how to address health promotion and prevention issues.

In the last two years, BIN has also been consulted by policy makers in the revising of health and physical education curricula and classroom material in Newfoundland and Labrador. Officials involved in curriculum revisions have taken seriously our warning of the dangers involved in physical educators using the BMI to assess their students. These officials have also followed our recommendations to avoid focusing on body measurements in a specific classroom resource book for physical education teaching. While the provincial government is very much concerned with obesity, unhealthy eating and low physical activity, many policy makers also want to 'do no harm' with regard to eating practices and body image. For government officials concerned with wellness, BIN's emphasis on self-esteem seems complementary to initiatives focused solely on healthy eating and on the increase of physical activity, which might explain why BIN was funded by the provincial government. But our work also raises some critical questions about the province's approach to the relation between health and weight issues. In the next section I examine how BIN's work raises critical questions about health and weight while also being limited by its own contradictions and ambiguities.

BIN's Uneasy Location: Clashing Frameworks in the Field of Health Promotion and Disordered Eating Prevention

BIN's work seems to 'add' to other initiatives funded by the provincial government because in some ways it shares the same psycho-behaviourial approach to health promotion. Since its inception BIN has been very much inspired by the Health Canada *Vitality* campaign, launched in 1991, and its focus on eating well, being active and, in particular, feeling good about oneself. The *Vitality* campaign emphasizes that individuals and families need to make good choices for themselves and change their behaviours if necessary. While self-esteem is an important addition to healthy eating and physical activity, it does not change the fact that the overall approach encourages personal responsibility and self-monitoring (MacNeill 1999).

The *Vitality* campaign fizzled in recent years due to insufficient funds; moreover, there were disagreements among federal health officials around promoting self-esteem which some considered 'too fuzzy' a concept and consequently the self-esteem and body image component of the message has been lost (Ellis 2007). Yet many organizations in Canada and elsewhere continue using this framework for heath promotion indicating its enduring appeal (Ellis 2007).

Like other organizations devoted to promoting a positive body image, BIN's approach may be hampered by its own contradictory and maybe irreconcilable assumptions. Moulding (2007) has studied a similar organization in Australia and found that its members attempted to promote critical social advocacy and individual responsibility at the same time, with the consequence that their social marketing approach undermined their critical perspective. BIN's adoption of the *Vitality* approach also clashes with its own critical socio-cultural approach and attempts at advocacy for social change. BIN's members also come from different standpoints in thinking about health promotion: some adopt a psycho-behavioural framework, while others come from a broader critical and feminist socio-cultural approach. For the latter, BIN's work should squarely challenge the province's current approach to individual lifestyle issues and 'healthy body weights'. Yet BIN has attempted to influence policy in part by working within the system's parameters. Like the feminist/critical researchers Larkin and Rice (2005), we plan to keep speaking up about issues of disordered eating, body inequity, culture, power, body diversity, body harassment and bullying in the province. To do so I would argue we need to clarify our own orientations to health promotion internally as a group and reflect on our own contradictions and limitations.

Divergent conceptualizations of health problems have different implications for health promotion. The expanding field of eating disorder prevention reflects the internal contradictions and dilemmas I have just discussed. Many studies and initiatives adopt a psycho-behavioural approach. For instance, a number of programs have been developed in attempts to prevent disordered eating, particularly among youth, in tandem with attempts to promote a positive body image for all, since unhealthy and disordered eating appear linked to high body dissatisfaction (Paxton 2002; Stice and Shaw 2002). Many initiatives attempt to prevent disordered eating among youth through an emphasis on improving young people's self-esteem via critical medical literacy and other critical skills, and through the management of stress (Levine and Piran 2004; Neumark-Sztainer 2002; O'Dea and Maloney 2000). Paxton (2002) recommends programs directed at late primary and early high-school ages as very important target groups. Most recently, researchers and activists have recommended prevention programs addressed simultaneously to individuals, their social environments and the larger community. For instance, McVey, Tweed and Blackmore (2007) propose an ecological prevention program for youth that involves public health employees, parents and teachers, as well as students, where adults as well as youth examine their own body and weight biases. These prevention initiatives advocate the critical deconstruction of cultural expectations of the gendered body and argue that boys' relation to the body must be examined as well as girls' (McVey et al. 2007; Paxton 2002).

Some researchers working within a psycho-behavioural perspective assert that one should work toward the prevention of obesity and eating disorders simultaneously. Neumark-Sztainer and her colleagues have attempted to bring together these two fields of research and interventions (Neumark-Sztainer 2002 and 2005; Neumark-Sztainer, Wall, Haines, Story, Sherwood and van den Berg 2007). Neumark-Sztainer (2002) acknowledges that there are differences between eating disorders as psychiatric diagnoses and obesity as a condition based on anthropometric measurements. Interestingly, though, she discusses how not only binge eating but also generally disordered eating (for instance dieting) may lead to obesity, a point also made by other scholars (Gaesser 2002). In their 2007 study on shared risks and protective factors for overweight and disordered eating in adolescents, Neumark-Sztainer and her colleagues found that a significant percentage of overweight girls engage in extreme weight-control measures. Ultimately these researchers propose that health promotion address both obesity and disordered eating by decreasing weight-related pressures and concerns for adolescents and for peers and adults in their environments. They end their article by writing:

> Support for a lifestyle that is based around healthful eating and physical activity behaviours, and not around weight per se, may prove to be more effective in decreasing the high prevalence of overweight youth, without leading to an increase in an unhealthy weight preoccupation and disordered eating behaviours.
>
> (Neumark-Sztainer et al. 2007: 367)

As I read this recent article by Neumark-Sztainer and her colleagues (2007) I was struck by the savvy ways in which the authors attempt to bring together researchers in divergent fields over the issue of weight related health within a psycho-behavioural framework. Ultimately, I feel that these researchers believe there is too much emphasis on weight concerns in health research as well as in people's everyday lives. It is both sensible and a delightful irony to suggest that less concern with weight is the most likely strategy to get rid of the 'excess' weight which is such a concern for obesity researchers.

The studies I just mentioned are important and well recognized. But a number of feminist and other critical scholars in the field have recommended going further and adopting a broader political and social approach to prevent disordered eating. For instance, some suggest that prevention initiatives address changes in girls' experience with adolescence and puberty (Larkin and Rice 2005; Levine and Piran 2004; Smolak 2004), and go beyond the notion of teasing to seriously examine the impact of sexual harassment (Smolak 2004), bullying and weight and culture based harassment (Larkin and Rice 2005) on young people's eating practices and their relations to the body. Critical scholars warn that even the best intentioned prevention campaigns may be reinforcing the dominant discourse of individual responsibility for body/health and do little to foster critical thinking (Moulding 2007). Feminist critical scholars put power and the culture of schools and other institutions at the centre of the analysis of disordered eating practices and their prevention. They warn that a narrow focus on thinness and body image issues fails to address other important matters, such as cultural differences, race, class and other power dynamics which shape eating and bodily experiences (Evans, Rich and Holroyd 2004; Larkin and Rice 2005). Feminist and other critical scholars also critique the biomedical approach of eating disorders professionals who analyze specific eating patterns and behaviors as mental illnesses affecting a minority of the population. By way of contrast, feminist and other critical scholars view dominant discourses of the healthy body as logically leading to widespread disordered eating and medically diagnosed eating disorders (Campos 2004; Gremillion 2002 and 2003; Malson 1998). Focusing on a minority population as pathological is different, and has different implications, from considering the global socio-cultural, economic and political contexts for widespread disordered eating in the general population.

Ultimately, I agree with Rice and Russell (2004) that critical thinking about all dimensions of power and health is required for research and interventions promoting body equity for all. From this consideration of the work of researchers and activists in the field of obesity prevention, I turn now to research on how youth make connections between health, disordered eating and the body.

YOUTH IN A QUANDARY: DEALING WITH WEIGHT CONTROL, FOOD AND THE SOCIAL ENVIRONMENT

Youth's Conflation of Health and Beauty

Recently, a number of researchers have examined how young people view and take up health promotion messages and dominant discourses of the ideal body (Burrows and Wright 2004; George and Rail 2005; Larkin and Rice 2005; MacDonald, Rodger, Abbott, Ziviani and Jones 2005; Rice 2007; Rich 2006; Rich, Holroyd and Evans 2004; Wills backet-Milburn, Grefory and Lawton 2006; Wright, O'Flynn and MacDonald 2006). A major finding in our research (Rail, Beausoleil, MacNeill, Burrows and Wright, 2003–6) is that Canadian youth conflate health, fitness and beauty.

Like young people in the Ottawa and Toronto regions (see Rail's chapter), the young people we talked with in Newfoundland and in New Brunswick defined both health and fitness as having a particular body shape and weight, and more specifically avoiding being fat, overweight or obese.

In their talk about health, the young people listed exercise, healthy fruits and vegetables and 'not being too overweight' as key aspects of good health. 'Being active,' or 'being in shape,' and 'not being fat' were equated and constantly brought up in the conversations. They saw a healthy body as a thin body, which, in turn, was an attractive body. One young person emphasized 'if you're healthy you're attractive'. For the young people who talked with us, 'not being fat' also allows one to live longer. For instance, in a small group discussion with young male immigrants, Strife answered the interviewer's question, 'What makes you concerned (about health)?', by saying, 'Umm . . . I don't want to go fat'. Chad added 'yeah', Greg offered, 'I want to grow old. I don't want to die at, like, 60', and Michael concluded, 'I would like to get old too'.

Young people's concerns seemed more about 'looking good' or 'not being fat' than about 'being healthy'. The various stories we heard about 'looking good' and 'being healthy' were profoundly shaped by dominant sexist, racist, heterosexist and ableist social relations and dominant discourses of beauty. However, while sharing in dominant discourses of beauty, there were variations among the young people about what 'looking good' means. For instance, a group of young people with physical disabilities first defined being healthy as 'keeping in shape' and 'not being too overweight'. As they spoke at length, however, they emphasized that health was about physical activity and most importantly physical strength and endurance, for both girls and boys. More than any other young people interviewed in Newfoundland and New Brunswick, this group saw physical strength as the key factor for health.

Int: What about you? What do you think a healthy person looks like?
C (boy): Like me (showing his muscles, laughter). That's strong. At home I always scoot around. I scoot around on the floor.
E (girl): I used to do that too.
C: It's some hard though. You try getting down and doing it.
E: Lifting your own weight is good. I find that it is really good for me especially because I find that if I'm not in my chair, I am on the floor and I have to lift myself up to move around. Lifting my own weight makes me stronger.
C: Do you scoot a lot?
E: Yeah.
C: I scoot up and down the stairs, up and down off my bed, up and down off the chair, and up and down off the couch and stuff.

Given the dominant ableist discourses of the healthy body, it is not surprising that the young people with physical disabilities would emphasize physical strength as crucial for good health. Yet for girls the emphasis on physical strength is potentially subversive, calling into question the definition of the ideal feminine body as weaker than the masculine body.

Young People's Critical Reflections

While largely adopting dominant discourses of health and the body, the young people also exercised agency and reflected critically about social processes. They were at times critical of dominant messages of health and the ideal body, which made for contradictory and complicated experiences in their every day lives. For instance, on the one hand, the participants in our study adopted the dominant discourse of individual responsibility for health as they emphasized healthy or unhealthy individual actions and lifestyles; most of the young people embraced the dominant notion of 'being fat' as bad for one's health. On the other hand, at times the young people in our study offered a critique of specific social environments as conducive to ill health. For example, recent immigrants (boys) offered a critique of food and eating practices in Canada:

> S: Well in Canada there are a lot of oversized people. My sister when she was in my home country (Liberia) she never used to eat a lot but when she came here all she did was eat, eat, and eat. My dad keeps telling her to stop eating because she will get fat but she won't and now she is getting big.
>
> G: You don't really eat more in terms of your meals it's just that you eat more like junk like chips and that . . . Yeah and then you start to put on weight and things like that . . . there is like junk everywhere. Like here in school and that it seems that everyone goes for the junk all the time and eat chips and that instead of a meal and like fast food . . . Home I ate so much fruits and vegetables a lot. In Colombia it is easy to get these foods, but like here some of the foods I ate are not even in the stores. People don't eat so many of those here I don't think.

This exchange is interesting as the second boy contradicts the first, saying people in Canada are not eating more per se but, rather, eat more bad food ('junk'). Recent immigrants from Columbia and Kenya emphasized that fruits and vegetables are expensive in Canada, in contrast to lower costs in their home countries. But unhealthy eating and obstacles to good nutrition particularly in schools were important topics for all youth who talked with us. The following exchange among a group of Muslim girls is typical of many discussions among our study participants.

> E: Well they could change the cafeteria food.
> M: Yeah it is so greasy all the time.

E: I mean they also serve things like French fries or say like pizza.

M: Yeah and the plate that they give it to you on is all full of grease it is so gross.

MAR: They could also make more gym classes and that.

MARI: Or sports teams too.

M: I find that one thing that is really interesting is like a bag of chips is like a dollar but then something more healthy would cost a lot more . . .

MAR: Yeah like vegetables cost like $5.

M: Yeah so maybe if they reduced the prices or whatever.

MAR: Healthy food costs a lot more than unhealthy food that is true.

M: Yeah that may also get people more interested into healthy foods.

S: I mean if the kids are not getting healthy foods and they do not eat them they get used to that. I mean then they will have a hard time changing that when they grow up.

E: I mean they will be more likely to eat junk food for sure or even fast food if they are used to eating that way all the time.

S: I mean physical activity needs to be important as well there is much more to being healthy than watching what you eat or whatever. You really need to be active as well.

In this excerpt, the young women both reinforce the dominant discourses of health as personal practices (eating and exercise) and challenge individualistic notions of health by emphasizing the wider social context. They indeed question public health discourses about food and physical activity that are inconsistent with their environments. The young people in our study also discussed a number of concrete obstacles to healthy eating and physical activity in schools: school structure, organization of the day at school; junk food in the cafeteria; high costs and lack of money; lack of time; pressure for school success; domestic chores; teasing and harassment; having the wrong body size and shape; gender bias and boys oriented sport programs; mixed gender physical activity classes; not enough gym or physical activity hours, limited choice of sports; and embarrassing fitness tests.

Though overwhelmingly thinking of 'being too fat' as a health danger, the young people also talked about the risk of ill health when people are 'too skinny' or overexercise. Participants considered girls who were too skinny at risk of, or already suffering from, anorexia nervosa. The young people we met did not talk about eating disorders among boys. For young men, being too skinny meant not having sufficient muscles. Clearly, young people observe those around them and have some knowledge of anorexia nervosa and this was reflected in the conversations they had with us about health. The young people who talked with us saw the occurrence of anorexia nervosa as the result of going too far in attempting to avoid the fat body. The young people also criticized beauty standards promoted in the media and popular culture as impossible to achieve in real life. Thus while readily adopting the dominant stance against the fat body, the young people in our study also offered some moments of critical consciousness about dominant discourses of the healthy body.

CONCLUSIONS

Purposively or inadvertently, campaigns to promote healthy eating and active living have the effect of reinforcing dominant discourses of the ideal body as lean and thin. Not surprisingly, fat hatred and discrimination against people deemed fat flourish. Researchers and activists working in the fields of eating disorders and disordered eating are told to consider 'the problem of obesity'. Even the authors of a recent article in a prestigious feminist journal (*Signs*) admonish feminist researchers for ignoring the health problems associated with obesity in favor of focusing on eating disorders such as bulimia and anorexia, which the authors characterize as affecting only a 'small minority of women' (Yancey, Leslie and Abel 2006: 426).

What can be done then to counter the disciplining of bodies through health discourses and regulatory practices? Organizations such as the Body Image Network (BIN) are attempting to counteract the dominant discourses but might be doing too little, not going far enough in their critique. Yet research with young people shows that the disciplining of the body is not quite complete. The young people we talked to for our research project tended to conflate health with beauty but they also at times reflected critically on their environments and saw dangers in pursuing thinness at all cost. Their narratives demonstrated that strong regulatory health mechanisms did not achieve a complete disciplining of young bodies. Young people's lack of power in shaping schooling and health promotion campaigns, and their lack of power in general, may ironically position them particularly well for critical thinking about concrete obstacles to health in people's everyday lives.

From a socio-cultural and critical perspective, I believe it is crucial to separate weight concerns from health issues; lifestyle has to take a back seat to most important broader social, economic and political determinants of health. But the reality of working with many health professionals invested in biomedical and psycho-behavioural approaches makes abandoning weight a challenge. Whether working in the fields of obesity or medically diagnosed eating disorders, most researchers and practitioners are associating specific anthropometric measurements with health or ill-health, albeit in different ways and for different reasons. Health professionals have powerful voices in shaping health policy campaigns and initiatives in schools and in the overall community. Contemporary healthist culture indeed configures body shape, size, and weight as the measure of both one's well-being and health. Those who create a panic about obesity reinforce disordered eating, while brandishing 'healthy eating' as one of their key messages. In this particular context, preventing disordered eating might well be an impossible task, but one worth attempting nonetheless. As a feminist researcher committed to social change, I want to believe that regulatory mechanisms, as subtle as they are, can be challenged, and that bodies can never be completely disciplined.

NOTES

1. The researchers thank the Social Sciences and Humanities Research Council of Canada for its generous support of this project.

REFERENCES

Burrows, L. and Wright, J. (2004) 'The Discursive Production of Childhood, Identity and Health', in J. Evans, B. Davies, and J. Wright (eds) *Body Knowledge and Control: Studies in the Sociology of Physical Education and Health*, London: Routledge.

Campos, P. (2004) *The Obesity Myth*, New York: Gotham Books.

Canadian Fitness and Lifestyle Research Institute (2007) 'Kids CAN PLAY-Bulletins', *Newfoundland and Labarador—Bulletin 1.1*, 20 December: retrieved 22 July 2008, from http://www.cflri.ca/eng/statistics/surveys/kidscanplay_bulletin1.php

Department of Health and Community Services (2002) *Strategic Health Plan for Newfoundland and Labrador*, St John's, Newfoundland: Department of Health and Community Services.

Department of Health and Community Services (2006) *Provincial Wellness Plan*, St John's, Newfoundland: Department of Health and Community Services.

Ellis, A. (2007) 'Presentations by policy makers: Ann Ellis, Health Canada', presented to the national symposium *Obesity and Eating Disorders: seeking common grounds to promote health*, Calgary, 5–6 November.

Evans, J. Rich, E. and Holroyd, R. (2004) 'Disordered eating and disordered schooling: what schools do to middle-class girls', *British Journal of Sociology of Education*, 25(2): 123–42.

Gaesser, G.A. (2002) *Big Fat Lies: The Truth About Your Weight and Your Health*, Carlsbad (CA): Gurze Books.

Gard, M. and Wright, J. (2005) *The Obesity Epidemic: Science, Mortality and Ideology*, London and New York: Routledge.

George, T. and Rail, G. (2005) 'Barbie Meets the Bindi: discursive constructions of health among young South-Asian Canadian women', *Women's Health & Urban Life*, 4(2): 45–67.

Gremillion, H. (2002) 'In fitness and in health: crafting bodies in the treatment of anorexia nervosa', *Signs*, 27(2): 381–414.

Gremillion, H. (2003) *Feeding Anorexia : Gender and Power at a Treatment Centre*, Durham and London: Duke University Press.

Larkin, J. and Rice, C. (2005) 'Beyond "healthy eating" and "healthy weights": Harassment and the health curriculum in middle schools', *Body Image*, 2: 219–32.

Levine, M.P. and Piran, N. (2004) 'The role of body image in the prevention of eating disorders', *Body Image*, 1: 57–70.

Macdonald, D., Rodger, S., Abbott, R., Ziviani, J. and Jones, J. (2005) '"I could do with a pair of wings": perspectives on physical activity, bodies and health from young Australian children', *Sport, Education and Society*, 10(2): 195–209.

MacNeill, M. (1999) 'Social Marketing, Gender and the Science of Fitness: A Case Study of ParticipACTION Campaigns', in P. White and K. Young (eds) *Sport and Gender in Canada*, Toronto: Oxford University Press.

McVey, G., Tweed, S. and Blackmore, E. (2007) 'Healthy schools—healthy kids: a controlled evaluation of a comprehensive universal eating disorder prevention program', *Body Image*, 4: 115–36.

Malson, H. (1998) *The Thin Woman: Feminism, Post-Structuralism and the Social Psychology of Anorexia Nervosa*, London and New York: Routledge.

Moulding, N.T. (2007) '"Love your body, move your body, feed your body": discourses of self-care and social marketing in a body image health promotion program', *Critical Public Health*, 17(1): 57–69.

Neumark-Sztainer, D. (2002) 'Integrating the prevention of eating disorders and obesity: feasible or futile?', *Preventive Medicine*, 34: 299–309.

Neumark-Sztainer, D. (2005) 'Can we simultaneously work toward the prevention of obesity and eating disorders in children and adolescents, *International Journal of Eating Disorders*, 38: 220–7.

Neumark-Sztainer, D., Wall, M., Haines, J., Story, M., Sherwood, N. and van den Berg, P. (2007) 'Shared risk and protective factors for overweight and disordered eating in adolescents', *American Journal of Preventive Medicine*, 33(5): 359–69.

O'Dea, J. and Maloney, D. (2000) 'Preventing eating and body image problems in children and adolescents using the Health Promoting Schools framework', *Journal of School Health*, 70(1): 18–21.

Paxton, J.S. (2002) *Research Review of Body Image Programs: An Overview of Body Image Dissatisfaction Prevention Interventions*, Melbourne, Victoria: Victorian Government Department of Human Services.

Rail, G. and Beausoleil, N. (2003) 'Introduction: health panic discourses and the commodification of women's health in Canada', in N. Beausoleil and G. Rail (eds) *Special Issue: Health Panic and Women's Health, Atlantis: A Women's Studies Journal*, 27(2): 1–5.

Rail, G., Beausoleil, N., MacNeill, M., Burrows, L. and Wright, J. (2003) *Canadian youth's constructions of health and fitness*, unpublished grant proposal, University of Ottawa and Memorial University.

Rice, C. (2007) '"Becoming the fat girl": Acquisition of an unfit identity', *Women's Studies International Forum*, 30: 158–74.

Rice, C. and Russell, V. (2004) 'Embodying equity: Creating a space for the body in equity education', *Orbit*, 34(1): 19–20.

Rich, E. (2006) 'Anorexic dis(connection): managing anorexia as an illness and an identity', *Sociology of Health and Illness*, 28(3): 284–305.

Rich, E., Holroyd, R. and Evans, J. (2004) '"Hungry to be Noticed": Young Women, Anorexia and Schooling', in J. Evans, B. Davies and J. Wright (eds) *Body Knowledge and Control: Studies in the Sociology of Physical Education and Health*, London and New York: Routledge.

Smolak, L. (2004) 'Body image in children and adolescents: where do we go from here?', *Body Image*, 1: 15–28.

Statistics Canada (2004) *Community Health Survey*, retrieved 28 January 2007, from http://www.statcan.ca/english/freepub/82-003-XIE/82-003-XIE2005003.pdf

Stice, E. and Shaw, H. (2002) 'Role of body dissatisfaction in the onset and maintenance of eating pathology: a synthesis of research findings', *Journal of Psychosomatic Research*, 53(5): 985–93.

Turner, B. (1996) *The Body and Society : Explorations in Social Theory*, London: Sage.

Turner, B.S. (1995) 'Aging and Identity: Some Reflections on the Somatization of the Self', in M. Featherstone and A. Wernick (eds) *Images of Aging: Cultural Representations of Later Life*, London: Routledge.

Walker Lowry, K., Sallinen, B.J. and Janicke, D.M. (2007) 'The effects of weight management programs on self-esteem in pediatric overweight populations', *Journal of Pediatric Psychology Advance Access*: retrieved 20 June 2007, from http://jpepsy.oxfordjournals.org.qe2a-proxy.mun.ca/cgi/reprint/32/10/1179

Wills, W., Backett-Milburn, K., Grefory, S. and Lawton, J. (2006) 'Young Teenagers' perceptions of their own and other bodies: a qualitative study of obese, overweight and "normal" weight young people in Scotland', *Social Science & Medicine*, 62: 396–406.

Wright, J. (2004) 'Post-structural Methodologies: The Body, Schooling and Health', in J. Evans, B. Davies, and J. Wright (eds) *Body Knowledge and Control: Studies in the Sociology of Physical Education and Health*, London: Routledge.

Wright, J., O'Flynn, G. and Macdonald, D. (2006) 'Being fit and looking healthy: young women and men's constructions of health and fitness', *Sex Roles*, 54(9–10): 707–16.

Yancey, A., Leslie, J. and Abel, E.K. (2006) 'Obesity at the crossroads: Feminism and public health perspectives', *Signs: Journal of Women in Culture and Society*, 31(2): 425–43.

8 Governing Healthy Family Lifestyles through Discourses of Risk and Responsibility

Simone Fullagar

INTRODUCTION

Within advanced liberal societies health promotion discourses are increasingly targeting the risk of obesity and other lifestyle diseases through schools, media campaigns and community programs. Australian initiatives have been aimed primarily at changing individual beliefs and behaviour related to 'risky' food consumption and physical activity, as well as the provision of programs and infrastructure (Headley 2004). Drawing on Michel Foucault's (1991) trajectory of thinking about biopower and more contemporary work that engages with risk (Lupton 1999; Rose 2007), this chapter critically considers how health promotion expertise works as a 'technology of power' to shape the conduct of family life. Coveney (2006: 161) argues that family lifestyle practices have become a significant site through which health is governed:

> With the focus of prevention very much on children, the home and the family are regarded as the safe haven for the pedagogical improvement of children's eating habits and the introduction of exercise regimes.

The discursive formation of the 'healthy lifestyle' in the 1960s can also be understood as part of a new politico-ethical terrain where family members are urged to exercise freedom via 'technologies of the self' organized around the prevention of 'risk' related to concerns about overweight and obesity (Coveney 2006; Foucault 1988). This chapter draws upon research with different kinds of families, and their stories offer a compelling critique of health lifestyle imperatives.

Rationalities of risk calculation, identification, prevention and management underpin an intervention logic focused on obesity that has become normalized within our growing 'health consciousness' (Crawford 2006). In particular, constructions of fatness via the Body Mass Index (BMI) position 'overweight' subjects as unhealthy, risky and costly citizens. Through such highly technocratic notions of health risk obesity has been constituted as a visible threat to individual and social wellbeing that requires 'urgent' political and policy action, rather than critical reflection on the possible social effects. The newly elected Australian Labor government's desire to weigh 4 year old children is one technique that is likely to generate a range of adverse effects, and affects, on the wellbeing of individuals and contribute to social divisions. The emergence of obesity risk as a central policy concern in Australia exemplifies Rothstein's (2006: 215) argument about the policy making processes of social institutions whereby 'we are no longer simply concerned with the governance *of* risk, but we are now in an era of governance *by* risk'.

Obesity related policy initiatives in Australia have quickly mobilized the authority of scientific, economic, psychological and social discourses to explicitly link risk with the moral imperative to promote 'healthy lifestyles' as a problem of individual choice and behaviour. A range of truth claims about economic savings, longevity and reduced illness, greater productivity and individual happiness, support the 'fight against obesity'. For example, the new *Eat Well, Be Active* (Queensland Government 2007) initiative brings together health, education and sport/recreation portfolios to promote particular kinds of physical activities and food consumption practices that are positioned as the risk reducing responsibility of individuals and families. Yet, despite the 'well intentioned' rationale of health promotion to improve population wellbeing we know little about the complex effects of linking the reduction of obesity risk with healthy lifestyle practices on citizens themselves. How do individuals and families experience risk and respond to health promotion discourses? How do they negotiate the healthy lifestyle imperative amidst the competing demands of everyday life, social inequalities and complex relationships?

In this chapter I take up these questions to critically consider the effects (and affects) of healthy lifestyle discourses on the everyday leisure practices of several Australian families who participated in a qualitative research project. In particular I am interested in how family members negotiate the public health imperative to 'eat well and be active' in light of the risks and pleasures that they experience when making everyday healthy lifestyle choices. While health promotion clearly targets 'risky' leisure practices related to food consumption and inactivity (too much television, fast food etc), there has been little reflection on pleasure as a significant affective dimension of wellbeing (Coveney and Bunton 2003; Fullagar 2002). Rethinking the meaning of pleasure requires us to move beyond commonplace assumptions that assume the 'potentially risky' bodies of individuals are simply biomedical or behavioural problems to be rationally measured and managed. Rather, the lived body can be better understood as a site of discursive struggle, as competing meanings of health and lifestyle decisions are made in relation to the material circumstances and relational contexts of families (Moulding 2007). In addition, there has been little exploration of the embodied effects of particular health promotion discourses in terms of generating feelings of shame, despair or disengagement, that can undermine wellbeing and exacerbate social inequalities and problematic responses to the body (Fullagar 2003; Rich and Evans 2005; Thirlaway and Heggs 2005).

To explore these issues in greater detail I analyse 'texts' from a current health promotion campaign alongside the texts produced from the interview transcripts of four different kinds of families living in suburban Queensland. The juxtaposition of these texts enables an examination of the different rationalities and affects that arise from the embodied experience of negotiating discourses about healthy lifestyles and risk (Fusco 2007; Wright 2004). This discursive approach also brings different registers of meaning into relation with each other and repositions different sources of authority (expert and lay) alongside each other (Game 1991; Hermes 1995). This type of analysis unsettles the power–knowledge relations that inform truths about health promotion, in particular the expert authority of policy and the assumed lack of expertise of individuals who, it is assumed, need to be 'better educated' about risk and benefit. The analysis of family repertoires of leisure and lifestyle practices offers a critique of the imperative within much health promotion material that urges individuals to adopt particular health practices, such as physical activity and food consumption, in order to reduce their risk of obesity related illnesses.

In the next section I analyse selected aspects of the text from the Queensland government's *Eat Well, Be Active* campaign that was distributed to each household during 2007 in a brightly coloured kit titled 'Your Life, Make the Most of it' (Queensland Government 2007). This kit consists of a sleeve with detailed pull out information sheets and celebrity photos (such as Australian tennis champion Pat Rafter) that specifically target adults and children (with titles such as 'active kids', 'bodyweight', 'family fun', 'activity guide' etc). I interweave these texts with contemporary ideas about the government of health as a means of identifying the tensions and contradictions that characterize the healthy lifestyle imperative.

MAXIMISING HEALTHY BODIES THROUGH RISK MINIMISATION

> Living a happier, healthier lifestyle comes naturally with eating well and being physically active . . . Being active combined with eating well helps maintain a healthy body weight.
>
> ('Your life, make the most of it', Queensland Government, 2007)

In this text from the *Eat Well, Be Active* campaign, healthy lifestyles come 'naturally' through the adoption of particular eating and activity practices that are tied to the achievement of a certain body weight and by extension happiness. Individuals are urged to embrace an ethos of health that seeks to 'maximize' their embodied capacities. Following Foucault's (Lemke 2001) work on the exercise of biopower in relation to the government of population health, Rose (2007) and others have begun to identify emerging discourses that articulate the production and maximisation of 'life itself'. Central to this shift is a reconfigured notion of the body beyond the focus of the clinical gaze towards a different somatic conception of subjectivity that visualizes life at the molecular level. Rose argues that a very different medical assemblage has taken shape through new techniques of government focused on ameliorating risk of illness where,

> The maintenance of the healthy body became central to the self management of many individuals and families, employing practices ranging from dietetics and exercise, through the consumption of proprietary medicines and health supplements, to self diagnosis and treatment.
>
> (Rose 2007: 10)

The self management of healthy lifestyles in advanced liberalism,[1] however, raises a key dilemma for State sponsored agencies that endeavor to 'govern at a distance' the freedom of citizens via moral prescriptions about how to live well (Dean 2007). State agencies cannot directly regulate or legislate so that individuals and families act in healthier ways. Instead a range of government and non-government agencies work in different ways to urge the population to exercise more responsibility for disciplining their own bodies and desires for 'unhealthy pleasures' in order to achieve moral selfhood through appropriate leisure choices. Tensions arise in relation to the individual freedom associated with leisure choices and the imperative to pursue particular activities that have value as 'risk reducing' strategies (Fullagar 2007). Minimizing health risks linked to lifestyle diseases becomes the rationale behind promoting active recreation and healthy eating as techniques for acting upon the (actual or potential) overweight body. The pleasure or meaning that one might derive from embodying recreation or food consumption are secondary concerns in an economy of risk structured through the metaphor of balancing energy 'inputs and outputs' (Gard and Wright 2005). This calculative logic is evident in the following text from the *Eat Well, Be Active* campaign that is accompanied by a photo of tennis player Pat Rafter,

> Getting the right balance between eating well and being active is the best way to maintain a healthy bodyweight and help to prevent serious illnesses like type 2 diabetes, cardiovascular disease, high blood pressure, kidney disease and some types of cancer.
>
> ('Your life, make the most of it', Queensland Government, 2007)

In this text there is an implicit moral value attached to acting on the body in a responsible, scientific mode through reference to a range of diseases, and more specific practices for 'building healthy bones, joints and muscles'. The text goes on to outline the benefits of healthy lifestyles in terms of the experiential dimensions of active living ('reducing feelings of stress and improving mental health, socialising opportunities') that embrace the ethic of lifestyle maximisation (Rose 1999) to get 'more out of life'. The figure of the healthy citizen implicit in this discourse is that of the 'responsible eater' (and by extension exerciser) (Coveney 2006) who is productive, entrepreneurial and works hard on the self-project of health. There are echoes of the flexible worker adapting to competitive market forces within this new mode of active living that is not particularly leisurely, relaxing or collaborative (Ericson and Doyle 2003). Individuals are required to work harder and 'invest' in themselves to modify their risky leisure choices to receive future benefits (longevity, reduced illness) from healthy lifestyles, regardless of mitigating social circumstances.

The focus on individualized health practices and risk reducing rationalities in the *Eat Well, Be Active* campaign denies the social relations of active living, the values and politico–ethical aspects of everyday experiences in homes, neighbourhoods, workplaces, schools and communities. This absence is curious given that the 'why be active' information sheet specifically identifies the 'contributing factors' (such as computers and car use) to inactivity and 'the rapid increase in obesity and other health problems'. There is little critical reference to the need to challenge workplace practices that contribute to work-life 'imbalances' and sedentary lifestyles, or questioning the ethic of consumption through which the meaning of modern life is mediated. Neither is there consideration of the possibility that alternative rationalities exist. For example, cycling may not be meaningful to the individual in terms of its capacity to alter metabolic rates but rather in terms of its perceived environmental benefits, networks of community or pleasurable physicality.

CONSUMPTION, HEALTHY LIFESTYLES AND THE SIGNIFICANCE OF AFFECT

Within the culture of consumption that is produced via the networks of global capital, individuals are urged to associate pleasure with acquiring, consuming and displaying consumer identities, despite often having limited material resources and/or time due to work, parenting etc (Bauman 2005; Crawford 2006). My own observation of the large numbers of weekend shoppers in suburban Queensland, after the introduction of Sunday trading several years ago, suggests that the culture of leisure consumption has intensified and weekend time available for active pursuits has come under increasing pressure. In response to individual 'time constraints', health promotion discourses mobilize techniques of calculating and measuring the temporal requirements of physical activity ('30 minutes a day for adults,

60 minutes for kids, 10 minute bouts'). Yet, these technocratic rationalities ignore the tensions between pleasure, desires to consume and disciplined healthy lifestyles that generate a range of emotions, or affects, that individuals and families have to constantly negotiate (Davidson, Bondi and Smith 2005). Despite their seemingly objective scientific claims about risk, health promotion discourses actually work to mobilize emotion, or affect, through 'fear' of bodily decline and 'guilt' about a lack of self-discipline or fitness (Bauman 2005; Furedi 1997). Parents, in particular, are urged to take up the active imperative to govern their own bodies and also as a means of inculcating good habits within children's bodies,

> Our actions as parents have a huge impact on the behaviour of our children. In fact, children of active parents are more active themselves. So it is very important for parents to get out there and set the example— show kids it's fun to be active and they'll be happy to be active too! Getting active together helps improve relationships.
>
> ('Get active together' information sheet, Queensland Government 2007)

Within this text is the enduring ideal of family togetherness that is refigured through 'health' as both serious responsibility and a source of fun; the family that plays together and eats well stays happily together (Miller 2000). In this sense, leisure is a site where families are 'responsiblized' and urged to assume the moral weight of addressing health issues as freely choosing lifestyle agents (Rose 1999). What is ignored here is the emotional tension that arises in modern family relations through the need to juggle expectations of togetherness with competing social demands related to work, leisure consumption, household labour and different individual interests/ needs. The emotional, or affective, aspect of lifestyle practices is shaped by the web of intimate and social relationships that mediate the decisions of individuals and families about the conduct of healthy citizenship. Yet, the power of affect tends to be under examined within the governmentality literature despite the growth of cultural and sociological theory in this area (Ahmed 2004; Bendelow 1998; Lupton 1998; Massumi 2002; Probyn 2005; Sedgwick 2003).

Theories of emotion, or affect, offer a different way of thinking through the body as a site of subjection that does not simply privilege self-conscious knowing or discursive regimes. Although there are ongoing debates about the differences between emotion and affect that generally fall along a sociological–biological continuum, post-structural perspectives acknowledge the impossibility of any conceptual–material divide. For example, by considering the relational context of what emotions 'do', Ahmed (2004: 4) explores how, 'emotions shape the very surfaces of bodies, which take shape through the repetition of actions over time, as well as through orientations towards and away from others'. Considering how individuals feel about 'being healthy' and what those feelings 'do' in relation to lifestyle choices can tell us much about how health is a negotiated and contested moral terrain in everyday life. As somatic selves we may well be urged to understand our embodied existence through the discourses of molecular science, but choices and desires are also mediated by relationships and emotions that connect us with each other. Emotions are profoundly relational; they shape our identities, as Ahmed (2004: 10) argues,

> So emotions are not simply something 'I' or 'we' have. Rather, it is through emotions, or how we respond to objects and others, that surfaces or boundaries are made: the 'I' and the 'we' are shaped by, and even take the shape of, contact with others.

To take this point further Massumi (2002) argues that different embodied affects move and disturb us; they exceed and escape the limits of rational knowing and thus 'make trouble' for the rationalist assumptions informing health promotion. Exploring the significance of affective experiences and relations is particularly important in the context of researching how families govern their own lifestyle choices and identities in relation to health expertise.

THE FAMILY LEISURE RESEARCH PROJECT

A qualitative study was undertaken to explore experiences of healthy lifestyles with four families that included seven parents and 14 children in lower-middle income suburbs of Brisbane. However, rather than presume this research method enabled access to unmediated truth about family life I acknowledge that the following representation is mediated by the interpretive process itself (Dupuis 1999). Families were recruited from community newspaper notices, email notices and fliers distributed through local networks, to talk about their 'leisure practices' rather than some narrowly defined notion of healthy lifestyle. The three members of the research team visited each family's home to conduct semi-structured individual interviews with seven adults, and combined or individual interviews with six children in late 2006. Participants were asked about all the different leisure practices undertaken as individuals and as a family (not just active pursuits), perceptions of healthy lifestyle issues and messages, what prevented them from engaging in leisure, risk issues and what changes they would like to see in their community. Transcripts of interviews were sent back separately to each participant in the family, including the children, and no changes were made by participants. A discursive analysis of the rationalities informing family repertoires of leisure, healthy lifestyles and risk was then undertaken (Rich and Evans 2005).

The following brief descriptions of the four different family backgrounds provide a glimpse into the everyday social context of their lives. Each family was given a pseudonym that suggests how they (and we) constructed a sense of identity through the leisure practices they valued. A range of family leisure experiences were identified and these also reflected common notions of family ideals in the literature; time spent being together, developing emotional connection, displaying family life publicly, purposively creating positive experiences and shared memories (Hallman, Mary and Benbow 2007; Shaw and Dawson 2001).

The Parks family can be characterized as middle-income, Anglo Celtic nuclear family with six children aged from 1 to 17 years old. They hold Christian beliefs, save to send their children to private schools and rent a two-story fibreboard house with a backyard in the middle suburbs of Brisbane. Father, Elvis 38, works full time in a white-collar job and mother Maree 37 has primary home duties with limited casual work. Daughters Clare 15 and Louise 11 were interviewed together.

The Rider family can be characterized as an Anglo Celtic, same-sex blended family who live in a rented house in a middle-income, inner suburban area of Brisbane. Melissa 29 is a mature age student with a daughter Jordan eight, from a previous relationship, and the other parent Kate 32 is employed full time. Melissa identified herself as previously having been obese for a number of years. Kate has a non-biological child (4 years) who does not reside at their home, but has regular visitation every second weekend for three to four days. Kate and Melissa have been living together for 1 year and identify their family as consisting of themselves and the two girls (Jordon was interviewed).

The Keepfit family consists of sole parent Kerry 49 and her four sons, of whom Harry 15 and Jack 10 (youngest) were interviewed. They live in a low-middle-income, outer suburban area of Brisbane in their own fibreboard home on a very large block with a pool. Their backyard is planted in native trees and shrubs, has a chicken pen and a makeshift archery range was set up at the time of the interview. Kerry is Anglo Celtic and works casually in education, she is divorced from the boys' father who lives an hour away and was not interviewed for the project.

The Karaoke family is an Anglo Celtic blended nuclear family that lives in a low-income outer suburban area of Brisbane in rented fibreboard housing. Dan, 39 has an illness that prevents him from working full time in his trade as a mechanic, while Barbara 38 undertakes home duties and struggles with the issues of sleep apnoea and overweight. They have two children, a teenage daughter 13 (not interviewed) with a serious neurological condition that caused rapid weight gain and sleep apnoea, and a younger son Scott aged 10.

The social biographical context of these families counters the depersonalized population focus of much health promotion research. Although we did not explicitly seek to recruit families experiencing weight related issues we found that three out of the four were trying to address this as a 'problem' in some way. To different degrees these three families viewed body size as a problematic reflection of their health status. As the following quotation from the 'Why be active?' information sheet, illustrates, the *Eat Well, Be Active* campaign reiterates this embodied relation between activity and eating in terms of the problem of maintaining normative weight as an indicator of health: 'Being active combined with eating well helps maintain a healthy bodyweight' (Queensland Government 2007).

The figure of the fat body is implicitly positioned in the *Eat Well, Be Active* campaign within a series of binary oppositions—healthy/unhealthy subjecthood, moral/immoral conduct, active/sedentary leisure, disciplined/undisciplined eating. These oppositions were also evident within the family interviews in terms of particular tensions produced through the desire to practice healthy lifestyles and the challenges of negotiating the complex relations of family life. All adult and child participants were familiar (to different degrees) with public health messages about eating well (fruit and vegetables, balanced diet) and being active (regular exercise, active choices). This 'health literacy' was also an articulation of their desire to embody healthy lifestyles and in this way they were 'ideal' neo-liberal subjects, positioning themselves as morally responsible citizens, despite often having limited material resources. Each family was dealing with health related issues in their attempt to transform aspects of their everyday lives, except for the Keepfit family whose sole parent Kerry, resisted expert advice to become healthier. Kerry felt she had always embraced 'hippie' ideals and healthy practices in her family life and felt that the obesity discourse was a 'panic' response.

AFFECT AND FAMILY DISRUPTION/CONNECTION

> Did you know that watching TV or DVDs, playing computer games and surfing the Net for more than two hours a day is associated with being overweight and poor fitness in adulthood? Reduce the risk and set limits of two hours a day max in front of the screen—unless it's homework!
>
> ('Teens and screens' information sheet,
> Queensland Government 2007)

The campaign as indicated in the quote above urges parents to regulate their children's 'passive leisure' (but not educational) pursuits to enable more time for activity that promises to reduce the risk of future obesity. However, for the Parks family playing video games together on the television was a favourite leisure pursuit that enabled enjoyable 'family time' (Daly 1996). Other family leisure pursuits were organized around a sense of shared identity such as going to local and city parks, 'we love doing stuff together, that's just the sort of family we are' (Maree Parks). While the

Parks did talk about the importance of a healthy lifestyle, concerns about father Elvis' overweight did not significantly shape their talk about their leisure time. Maree and Elvis described themselves as trying to make healthier food choices (gendered as Maree's responsibility when cooking) but their physical activity pursuits with the six children remained unchanged. Maree's identification of fad diets (mentioned in relation to another family who follow a strict reduced carbohydrate diet with their young children) as 'extremist' also suggested some resistance to taking up discourses about the problematic body that would position her children's bodies as sites of obesity risk.

Rather than the body being viewed fearfully as a site of risk, the Parks family identified mental health or mind–body relations, particularly in terms of their teenage daughter's depression, as a more significant area of risk. Hence, it was not surprising that they articulated the importance of leisure in terms of facilitating positive emotional relationships and countering some of the negative affects related to depression (shame, despair, meaninglessness). Amidst the busyness of the Parks family life, shared leisure practices were sought out as a means of 'doing' emotional connectedness and thus family identity (Ahmed 2004). This finding offers a challenge to the way health promotion discourses tend to assume an instrumental notion of the body as an eating and exercising machine, rather than a medium of thinking and feeling that exists within the relational bonds of family life.

In contrast to the normative context of the Parks family, the same-sex blended Rider family talked about the negative emotional impact of inadequate same-sex custody laws on their sense of wellbeing and child access. The Riders also experienced emotional struggles with overweight and finding ways to develop healthier and enjoyable lifestyle practices. Melissa described herself as a sporty person and yet she became, in her words, 'obese' as a sole parent, and this was compounded by her own struggle with emerging sexual identity issues.[2] Her experience contrasts with the instrumental rationalities informing health promotion discourses that tend to ignore the embodied nature of 'risk' that is shaped by social circumstances. For example, the body is positioned as an object of calculation and intervention,

> Check your body mass index (on the chart) . . . these guides can help determine if you are at risk of illnesses such as type 2 diabetes and heart disease . . . If you're concerned or unsure about your bodyweight or BMI, visit your doctor . . . another way to measure your weight-related health is with a tape measure . . . Aim for a healthy lifestyle. This takes into account your physical, mental and social wellbeing.
> ('Do you have a healthy bodyweight and measure up' information sheets, Queensland Government 2007)

Melissa recounted how she was told by a doctor that she was obese and faced increased risks to her health. She described this as having little impact on her desire to change her lifestyle because she already 'knew' this. What altered her desire to embody a different lifestyle was an experience of risk (heart thumping, unable to run), a wish to create better opportunities for her daughter Jordon and the support of her new partner Katie. The Rider family made major lifestyle changes (more cycling, deliberate eating out decisions) and Melissa lost a large amount of weight, although she maintained this was an ongoing struggle. Part of the struggle was dealing with the emotional dynamics of being a newly formed lesbian family, rather than some notion of a lack of self-discipline in relation to health regimes. Melissa talked about the emotional dimension of performing 'family' in their leisure time, 'We go out as a family. If that means Katie and I are holding hands, we're holding hands. If we choose to have a cuddle in the park, we have a cuddle in the park. Like, we don't care.' The 'doing' of emotion through the Rider family's leisure was shaped by their desire to 'display' (belonging, pride, love etc) and thus create a non-normative identity within the normative context of public spaces (playing in parks, cycling, shopping, attending festivals etc) (Finch 2007). Yet, as other research also identifies (Gabb, 2005) the normative legal and cultural context of 'family life' undermined the Rider family's sense of recognition, entitlement and visibility, which contributed to their feelings of uncertainty and anxiety.

Engaging in gay and lesbian specific leisure events also helped the Riders feel less 'othered' by heteronormativity, as Melissa said, 'its good for our daughters to see that, to say that its normal, it happens. The way our family is . . . it's not a one-off . . . that there are others out there'. Through this experience we can see how the emotional terrain of family life is mediated by social forces that shape normative and non-normative identities, and thus health and leisure opportunities, in terms of difference structured around sexuality, gender, ethnicity and class. The struggle to achieve 'health' was a source of great tension for the Riders as the very 'doing' of family life is itself 'risky' and the presumption of parental rights or 'choice' as the basis for stability is precarious. Along with the neglect of emotion, health promotion discourses marginalize diverse family identities and the meaning of leisure by ignoring how risk is experienced differently within the social order. As other sociological research has indicated family decisions about leisure pursuits and food are intimately bound up with class cultures and gendered responsibilities that construct risks to children's wellbeing in very different ways (Vincent and Ball 2007). I return to the relationship between family leisure repertoires and risk later in the chapter.

The Karaoke family also experienced multiple health issues that included mother Barbara's sleep apnoea and her daughter's neurological condition that exacerbated appetite, and both were struggling with overweight issues. The father, Dan, had a chronic illness that prevented him from working full-time and there was some concern over son, Scott's future weight gain (he was not evidently overweight but there were concerns he might be one day). Managing the emotional demands of family life along with health issues was described by Barbara as hard work, 'I think it is like my energy is down and the . . . children need me at certain times . . . I get a bit cranky and a bit grumpy and I might say something that I should not have said'. Barbara used strategies to create leisure time and space to renew her energy, such as shopping for bargains ('it is like a sport for me') and relaxing in the backyard. Despite her strategies and good intentions it was a constant struggle to develop a healthy family lifestyle both financially and emotionally, 'I mean food is not cheap either, especially healthy food'. Barbara talked about her own fear of having a heart attack, and her guilty pleasure in consuming 'unhealthy' foods when stressed, through a discourse of moral (and gendered) responsibility for family wellbeing,

> the obesity on top of that, that really stresses me out at the moment, it has for a long time . . . trying to keep the weight down with my son and trying to keep my daughter on a plateau and myself, I mean I have been up and down . . . I am usually her guide, I might have a bit of a snack attack, I feel guilty for it, I will go into my room I will not do it in front of her or anything like that because she has a problem with managing it herself.

For Barbara her embodied experience of health risk and gendered sense of responsibility for her daughter also shifted her desire to change aspects of the family lifestyle. They 'worked' at modifying eating habits and encouraging their children to be active everyday. This effort to be healthy was contrasted with the pleasures associated with family leisure pursuits that were inclusive and enabled children to feel good about themselves without the moral imperative to be 'health improving',

> We go to my best friend's house . . . and we usually have a BBQ or just have a sing along. She has the microphones and I have the amp, with all the children, nieces and nephews . . . We are karaoke junkies . . . What do I enjoy about karaoke? . . . trying to help people with self confidence, they might feel like they can not sing but . . . if they need help with their singing, you know from a young age to the elderly I will get up there and I'll say come on let's give it a go. Like there is no judgement.

The importance of family leisure time for 'doing' emotional connection was reiterated by the Karaokes in relation to the class related issues their children had experienced (bullying in sport, violence, lack of confidence, poor body image, disconnection from peers, depression and anger issues). Barbara articulated a sense of 'doing family leisure' that was central to her own 'successful' subjecthood as a lower income mother and countered her sense of failure in relation to weight. She valued connectedness and affirming experiences for her children rather than the (middle-class) pursuit of healthy lifestyles as a means of maximising their life chances or opportunities for success. When asked what was important to her about family leisure Barbara mentioned time for,

> Laughing, because my daughter faces a lot of depression, up and down mood swings and my son's anger management. Laughing, to actually get on well together it makes me sort of feel more like a mother . . . you feel more worthy that you are there, I mean I should know myself that my children always love me . . . but it makes you feel a lot better within yourself because they appreciate who you are and then they get along well themselves, they behave themselves.

This narrative points toward the need for health promotion to further understand the gender and class dynamics of family life and how emotional tensions and pleasures are negotiated in relation to what constitutes 'well-being' rather than a more narrowly defined notion of health. For Barbara, leisure time together created an important space to create emotional connectedness because of,

> Anxiety, anxiety is another one we all face I think . . . my son will come up and say I am not feeling well. We might go for a walk it might be excess energy maybe from sugars that he has eaten or something like that, he might want to get out and get it out of his system we will go for a walk or have a chat about it or I might to need to spend time with my daughter or my husband . . . to have that time together, just to talk.

Dan (father) also thought that family leisure time created better communication between parents and children which helped them manage dangers, 'they communicate a lot better than most of the children on the street . . . which is really important around here because of the really, really, high number of drug users'. Dan raises the issue of risks, fears and dangers, other than those related to health, that significantly shape family decision-making about children's leisure pursuits and parental responsibilities. As described below, fear figured as a dominant emotion in the lives of the families who were constantly negotiating 'risk' in their everyday social situations. Healthy lifestyle discourses not only privilege rationality over emotion in their construction of family life, but also health risk over other kinds of dangers. In this way, they fail to engage with the complex and shifting meanings of health and wellbeing, risk and pleasure that shape diverse family lives.

RISK AND FAMILY FEARS

> Organize an active family adventure: explore a national park—camp or hike and pack a healthy picnic lunch; spend an afternoon at the beach; get on some bikes and explore your local area; walk, cycle or

use public transport instead of the car as a low cost, fun way to get the family more active.

('Get active together' information sheet,
Queensland Government 2007)

The affective power of fear to curtail children's leisure pursuits is also something that health promotion discourses tend to ignore in relation to risk. All the families interviewed in our research identified a range of dangers and employed particular risk management strategies to manage these 'threats' to children's wellbeing. Maree Parks talked explicitly about the need for surveillance as she liked to know 'where they are and what they're doing all the time'. Kerry Keepfit created her own private adventure playground on her large block of land where her sons could ride motorbikes, swim and kick balls around in close proximity to her. She was less concerned about her sons' safety as they got older and were able to get around independently. The Parks children were not allowed to ride their bikes on the street without adult supervision, while friends and social events (parties) were thoroughly screened by parents to ensure safety, 'particularly for the older girls'. Like other research has found, mobile phones were a common risk management strategy that enabled families to maintain contact with children beyond their direct supervision (Backett-Milburn 2004).

For the Karaoke family living in a poorer community with predominantly public housing, identifying and negotiating risk was part of everyday life. They described abductions, paedophiles living in the next street, indecent exposure on local bike paths and violence, which shaped the risk contours of public leisure spaces and directly affected what Dan allowed the children to do: 'it keeps them away from the park and I do not let them go out after dark . . . I tend to keep them paired up with someone if they go out . . . so that there is always someone to make plenty of noise'. Although Barbara knew that the police patrolled the bike paths she also expressed a deep uncertainty about the children's present and future freedom as 'it is quite difficult knowing what is out there'. Furedi (1997) argues, in a somewhat alarmist fashion, that the culture of fear leads to an inability to act and unwillingness to take risks. Yet, in this research families were constantly calculating the risk of moral and physical harm and the benefits of participating in family or individual leisure pursuits. Melissa Rider talked about how they were managing risk in relation to their young daughters,

> at this age we are just instilling some stuff about the foundations and building up to what sort of risks there could be in society as they grow older . . . it all comes down to leisure activities . . . Things kind of happen to you when you go out. You're doing stuff, whether its personal safety or realising that some activities that you do may be more dangerous than others or . . . Like rock-climbing, there are things that you know, steps that you need to take to prevent injury.

Leisure in this sense is inherently risky which means pleasure and danger have to be constantly evaluated, taught and negotiated by adults who facilitate children's experiences.

In contrast to the notion that physical activity is a 'natural' part of healthy lifestyles, this research suggests that leisure choices have become an emotionally intensified and complex aspect of family life. Children's autonomous play or leisure was no longer considered to be a time of freedom (often referred to in relation to their own childhoods) and unregulated exploration, and parents desired safer options in their local communities (e.g., supervized recreation centres, intergenerational sport competitions where the whole family could play, better transport etc). Family decision making about health and leisure was marked by tensions between the desire for safety and the desire to engage in pleasurable individual and family pursuits that were a valued source of emotional wellbeing (although often perceived in different ways by children and adults). Whether these 'risks' are real or perceived is beside the point, as the construction of risk shapes how families make decisions about how they spend their leisure time together or by themselves,without parent supervision. This in turn, illustrates what emotions can 'do' to prevent or enable family participation in healthy lifestyles.

Although health promotion discourses are underpinned by rationalist claims about educating and improving health awareness, they also seek to act upon the body and change the way individuals behave, interact and feel about food and physical activity. The text below assumes that the language of risk reduction is the motivating force that will sustain healthy lifestyle practices, while the stories of participants indicate a far more complex range of meanings.

> The gradual weight regain after initial weight loss is very common, and sometimes unavoidable. But keep up the good eating and physical activity to help reduce risk of serious illnesses.
>
> ('Keep up the good work' information sheet,
> Queensland Government 2007)

Risk discourses work to mobilize emotion or affect as they attempt to shape how we conduct ourselves as active, responsible healthy subjects. Despite the seemingly neutral language of science that is deployed in health messages about reducing lifestyle risks, affect is evoked through fears about illness, incapacity and death as well as the pleasures of family fun. Guilt also arises in relation to body size, appearance and parental decision making about children's wellbeing, while anger, frustration and despair can arise from the impossible demands of managing one's own, or one's family's health, as a rational, self resourced project. Yet, within the literature there is little research that explores how people, as embodied subjects, negotiate and produce meaning about healthy lifestyle practices in the complex socio-cultural, economic and political conditions of advanced liberalism. Rose (1999) identifies new technologies of government that work via the 'calculated administration of shame' and this has resonance for thinking about the significance of affect in obesity related health promotion initiatives. Not participating in normative healthy lifestyle regimes or being positioned as an unhealthy body is likely to generate shame for families (with different effects on parent and children) in public settings and private negotiations. The powerful effects of shame, as evidenced in the ongoing struggles of the research participants, ironically undermines the exercise of autonomy and responsibility that is assumed to freely exist as the basis for family decision making about health and leisure. Shame also generates feelings of failure for families that may further strain relationships and exacerbate the blame apportioned to individuals for their circumstances (Ahmed 2004).

CONCLUSION

The dominance of scientific and behavioural discourses in health promotion has contributed to a biomedical notion of the body as both the object of risk and the subject of risk reduction. This search for the truth in evidence based approaches and epidemiological calculation paradoxically ignores how individuals embody everyday leisure and health practices in the process of governing themselves within family relations. Importantly, meaning about healthy lifestyle practices needs to be understood as relational and constituted between people whose identities are marked by class, gender, ethnicity, sexuality, age, religion and disability. These social markers of identity work in complex ways to shape the conduct of self, and hence, the exercise of 'responsible freedom' through healthy lifestyle choices in advanced liberalism (Rose 2007). The figure of the 'responsible eater and exerciser' was evident in family stories that articulated a desire to practice healthy lifestyles in relation to active leisure pursuits (Coveney 2006). Yet, most families also valued non-active leisure pursuits (karaoke, computer games, watching films etc) because they created opportunities for 'doing' emotional connection that, in turn, created the positive feeling of 'family life'. Pleasurable time spent pursuing fun, laughter, letting go and just hanging out together was contrasted with the moral imperative to be continuously working to improve one's health through instrumental and rational calculations of risk and benefit. Women in particular identified a gendered difference in terms of the responsibility for undertaking the emotional work that informs the relational basis of family life and also the conduct of healthy lifestyle practices (planning meals, organising activities, negotiating with others, managing time etc). The family stories in this research stand in stark contrast to health promotion discourses that assume leisure and healthy lifestyle practices are 'naturally' occurring and somehow separate from the relational and emotional meaning of family life.

Different family formations and identifications also add to the complexity of understanding how individuals make choices alone, in relation to significant others and within the context of their communities. Health promotion acknowledges the importance of social and physical environments. Yet, little consideration is given to how diverse families have to negotiate a range of discourses that often work to marginalize and shame their identities through a kind of health moralism aimed at the 'fat, lazy, undeserving, irresponsible, abnormal' (Crawford 2006). If we are to critically consider the effects, and affects, of health promotion discourses on family life then we need to consider how non-normative families face an intensification of certain affects (such as shame) (Ahmed 2004). As the stories of participants demonstrate these affects can undermine a family's capacity to negotiate risky environments and hence their ability to conduct healthy lifestyle practices that are premised on white, middle class, heterosexual norms and material conditions.

Risk figured as a central motif in the leisure and health repertoires of all families in this study. Healthy lifestyle decisions were negotiated in relation to the perceived risks of moral and physical harm to children engaging in public leisure spaces, and the benefits derived from their independent participation. To understand how risk is lived, constructed and negotiated we need to situate the healthy lifestyle decisions of families (about children's or collective activities) within the broader context of discourses that connect leisure, health and risk. As the Rider family indicated, leisure practices are inherently risky in that children and adults have to negotiate both positive and negative dangers in order to participate in public life. In contrast to the argument put forth by Furedi (1997) that risk discourses lead to inaction, families in this study were actively engaged in calculating risks and benefits, pleasure and discipline, emotional connection and instrumental activity, autonomy and togetherness. Risk rationalities formed a significant part of the discursive terrain that shaped the conduct of healthy family lifestyles. However, they were intertwined with the embodied, affective and relational aspects of family life, and hence, advanced liberal practices of self-government. To conclude, this chapter has argued for a more critical approach to health promotion that examines the social forces that shape healthy lifestyle practices in relation to the effects, and affects, of policy imperatives on the lives of individuals and populations.

NOTES

1. Advanced liberalism is distinguished from the broader term neo-liberalism to indicate the specific liberal style of government and rationalities that produce notions of democratic freedom. Dean (2007: 192) identifies key characteristics such as globalised economic relations, individualised risk management and a belief in the supercession of national sovereignty.
2. I am not implying here that non-heterosexual identities or obesity are essentially problematic. Rather that this participant identified her own complex

negotiation of dominant discourses about identity that affected her sense of self and well-being.

REFERENCES

Ahmed, S. (2004) *The Cultural Politics of Emotion*, Edinburgh: Edinburgh University Press.

Backett-Milburn, K. (2004) 'How children and their families construct and negotiate risk, safety and danger', *Childhood*, 11(4): 429–47.

Bauman, Z. (2005) *Liquid Life*, Cambridge: Polity Press.

Bendelow, G.A.W.S. (ed.) (1998) *Emotions in Social Life: Critical Themes and Contemporary Issues*, London: Routledge.

Coveney, J. (2006) *Food, Morals and Meaning: The Pleasure and Anxiety of Eating*. London: Routledge.

Coveney, J. and Bunton, R. (2003) 'In pursuit of the study of pleasure: implications for health research and practice', *Health*, 7(2): 161–79.

Crawford, R. (2006) 'Health as a meaningful social practice', *Health*, 10(4): 401–20

Daly, K. (1996) *Families and Time: Keeping Pace in a Hurried Culture*, London: Sage.

Davidson, J., Bondi,L. and Smith, M. (eds) (2005) *Emotional Geographies*, Hampshire: Ashgate.

Dean, M. (2007) *Governing Societies: Political Perspectives on Domestic and International Rule*, Maidenhead: Open University Press.

Dupuis, S. (1999) 'Naked truths: towards a reflexive methodology in leisure research', *Leisure Sciences*, 21(1): 43–64.

Ericson, R. and Doyle, A. (eds) (2003) *Risk and Morality*, Toronto: University of Toronto.

Finch, J. (2007) 'Displaying families', *Sociology*, 41(1): 65–81.

Foucault, M. (1988) 'Technologies of the Self' in L. Martin, H. Gutman and P. Hutton (eds) *Technologies of the Self: A Seminar with Michel Foucault*, London: Travistock.

———.(1991) 'Governmentality' in G. Burchell, G. Gordon and P. Miller (eds) *The Foucault Eeffect: Studies in Governmentality*, Hemel Hempstead: Harvester Wheatsheaf.

Fullagar, S. (2002) 'Governing the healthy body: Discourses of leisure and lifestyle within Australian health policy', *Health: an interdisciplinary journal for the social study of health, illness and medicine*, 6(1): 69–84.

———.(2003) 'Governing women's active leisure: The gendered effects of calculative rationalities within Australian health policy', *Critical Public Health*, 13(1): 47–60.

———.(2007) 'Governing healthy families: Leisure and the politics of risk' in M. Casado-Diaz, S. Everett and S. Wilson (eds) *Social and Cultural Change: making space(s) for leisure and tourism*, Eastbourne: Leisure Studies Association, 98: 67–78.

Furedi, F. (1997) *The Culture of Fear: Risk Taking and the Morality of Low Expectation*, London: Cassell.

Fusco, C. (2007) '"Healthification" and the promises of urban space: A textual analysis of place, activity, youth (PLAY-ing) in the city', *International Review for the Sociology of Sport*, 42(1): 43–63.

Gabb, J. (2005) 'Lesbian m/otherhood: Strategies of familial–linguistic management in lesbian parent families', *Sociology*, 39(4): 585–603.

Game, A. (1991) *Undoing the Social: Towards a Deconstructive Sociology*, Milton Keynes: Open University Press.

Gard, M. and Wright, J. (2005) *The Obesity Epidemic: Science, Morality, and Ideology*, Oxford: Routledge.

Hallman, B., Mary, S. and Benbow, P. (2007) 'Family leisure, family photography and zoos: Exploring the emotional geographies of families', *Social and Cultural Geography*, 8(6): 871–88.

Headley, S. (2004) 'Local initiatives: Background notes on obesity and sport in young Australians', *Youth Studies Australia*, 23(1): 42–6.

Hermes, J. (1995) *Reading Women's Magazines: An Analysis of Everyday Media Use*, Cambridge: Polity Press.

Lemke, T. (2001) 'The birth of bio-politics: Michel Foucault's lecture at the Collège de France on neo-liberal governmentality', *Economy and Society*, 30(2): 190–207.

Lupton, D. (1998). *The Emotional Self*, London: Sage.

——.(1999) *Risk and Sociocultural Theory*, Cambridge: Cambridge University Press.

Massumi, B. (2002) *Parables for the Virtual: Movement, Affect, Sensation*, London: Duke University Press.

Miller, L. (2000) 'Family togetherness and the suburban ideal', *Sociological Forum*, 10(3): 393–418.

Moulding, N. (2007) '"Love your body, move your body, feed your body": Discourses of self-care and social marketing in a body image health promotion program', *Critical Public Health*, 17(1): 57–69.

Probyn, E. (2005) *Blush: Faces of Shame*, Sydney: University of New South Wales.

Queensland Government (2007) *Eat Well Be Active Campaign*, Brisbane: Queensland Government, retrieved 22 July 2008, from www.eatwellbeactive.qld.gov.au/

Rich, E. and Evans, J. (2005) '"Fat ethics"—The obesity discourse and body politics', *Social Theory & Health*, 3: 341–58.

Rose, N. (1999) *The Powers of Freedom: Reframing Political Thought*, Cambridge: Cambridge University Press.

——.(2007). *The Politics of Life Itself: Biomedicine, Power and Subjectivity in the Twenty-First Century*, Princeton: Princeton University Press.

Rothstein, H. (2006) 'The institutional origins of risk: a new agenda for risk research', *Health, Risk and Society*, 8(3): 215–21.

Sedgwick, E.K. (2003) *Touching, Feeling: Affect, Pedagogy, Performativity*, Durham, NC: Duke University Press.

Shaw, S. and Dawson, D. (2001) 'Purposive leisure: Examining parental discourses on family activities', *Leisure Sciences*, 23(4): 217–31.

Thirlaway, K. and Heggs, D. (2005) 'Interpreting risk messages: Women's responses to a health story', *Health, Risk and Society*, 7(2): 107–21.

Vincent, C. and Ball, S. (2007) '"Making up" the middle-class child: Families, activities and class dispositions', *Sociology*, 41(6): 1061–77.

Wright, J. (2004) 'Post-structural methodologies: The body, schooling and health' in J. Evans, B. Davies and J. Wright (eds) *Body Knowledge and Control: Studies in the Sociology of Physical Education and Health*, London: Routledge.

9   Pedagogizing Families through Obesity Discourse

Lisette Burrows

INTRODUCTION

Mission-On Not a religious phenomenon, nor a space odyssey, but rather, the catch-all title of the New Zealand government's 67 million dollar fat-busting regime, rolled out in 2007. In a context where obesity is heralded as the most pressing health concern of our age (Campos 2004; Campos, Saguy, Ernsberger, Oliver and Gaesser 2006; Gard and Wright 2005), nothing short of a 'mission' will do, say the instigators of this wide-sweeping package of 10 initiatives targeting the eating habits, physical activity patterns and environments of all New Zealanders (Clark 2006). As is the case with most health initiatives, in *Mission-On* early intervention is represented as the key to unlatching a lighter future. And, as has perennially been the case, families are positioned centrally in the governmental gaze.

In this chapter I specifically examine the array of disciplinary and normalizing practices obesity discourse generates in and around the home and the family. I interrogate these practices for the meanings they construct not only about what constitutes a good and healthful family but also for the kinds of messages conveyed about the kinds of bodies and selves that matter. My focus is not *Mission-On* per se, but rather how state power, as represented in packages like *Mission-On*, operates through what Foucault (1977) would term a diffuse set of technologies to not only govern the actions of families but also constitute families' understanding of themselves as viable, good and healthful units within a citizenry where 'fat' is an anathema.

One way to theorize these diffuse technologies is to think of them as biopedagogies, as techniques deployed as part of 'the art and practice of teaching of "life"' (Harwood in this collection). As Harwood points out in Chapter 2 of this book, using biopedagogies as an orienting theoretical concept draws attention to both the pedagogies directed to an individualized body as well as to the 'species' body. Thus, while describing what these packages and resources *are* is of some import, it is what they *do*, what instructions they provide on 'how to live', what they produce in the way of family relationships, normalized bodies, dispositions towards self and others, what they assume and what they preclude in terms of knowledge about the health of populations that is this chapter's main focus. How do packages like *Mission-On* help families assemble themselves into subjects? How does a power 'that appears life conserving' (Harwood—see Chapter 2 of this book) act on the actions of families and how may families in turn take up and resist the modes of subjectification and visions of the good, functional, life conserving and healthful family engendered by and through obesity discourse? How do families learn to self-govern and manage their lives in ways that render them intelligible families in obesity discourse? And what happens to those who can't or won't? As Foucault contends, '[t]o understand power in its materiality, its day to day operation, we must go to the level of the micropractices, the political technologies in which our practices are formed' (Dreyfus and Rabinow 1982: 185).

The expansion of techniques for ordering, managing, classifying and controlling populations that Foucault (1991) refers to as biopower is especially salient in any consideration of how and why the family is construed as so pivotal in obesity discourse. As Harwood (see Chapter 2 of this book) attests, biopower emphasizes the protection of life, and regulation of the body-foci that cohere with the discourses of 'protection' that have, since the establishment of 'childhood' as a category contoured the way adults conceive of their role in the lives of children (Archard 1993; Aries 1962; James and James 2004; Woodhouse 2004). That is, throughout history a view of childhood as a time of innocence and of vulnerability has featured prominently in popular discourse on good parenting, in the disciplinary texts of developmental psychology and in the resources that guide child development professionals (Bird 1994; Burman 1991; Mayall 1996 and 1998; Walkerdine 1984; Wyn and White 1997). As young and potentially vulnerable members of society, adult responsibilities lie in the protection of children from risks associated with phenomena like obesity. The risks are those potentially incurred through living in an 'obesogenic' environment, but importantly, in the case of obesity, risks linked to children's own propensities to unpredictably engage in unhealthful behaviours. A discourse of protection then, both establishes a rationale for state intervention in the lives of families and also a way of understanding *why* parents themselves may respond to health imperatives in ways that at times, appear at odds with what would 'normally' constitute 'good parenting'.

EXPERT TESTIMONY

Foucault (1977) maintains that scientific disciplines generate particular kinds of knowledge purveyed by experts that individuals draw upon to make sense of themselves as human subjects. This knowledge is also used to regulate populations, or as Foucault would term it, 'man-as-species' (Foucault 2003: 242). Although well rehearsed by others (Gard and Wright

2005) it is worth briefly reiterating the key themes of the expert childhood obesity testimony found in newspaper and tabloid reportage prior to analyzing the kinds of individualizing and 'massifying' (Foucault 2003: 243) practices that are linked to it.

Analysis of newspaper coverage in the latter 6 months of 2006 yielded a surfeit of commentary on children, parents and families in general with three notable trends emerging in the reportage. First, I noted the representation of children of younger and younger ages as both sources of and potential solutions to the obesity problem and an escalating panic about the *pace* at which children (and in some cases, infants) are getting fatter. As New Zealand's Prime Minister puts it:

> Unless something changes, the current generation of New Zealand children may very well be the first to die at a younger age than their parents . . . This issue is potentially the greatest single threat to the health of New Zealand families, and our biggest public health challenge.
>
> (Clark 2006)

Bolstered by scary statistics, emotive language and represented with a certainty that belies the shaky empirical foundations upon which most of the claims are premised, readers are left in no doubt that obesity *is* a major problem for all children virtually everywhere and that unless we take action now our lives and lifestyles will be severely threatened.

Drawing on developmental discourses that cast early intervention as a crucial fat-busting tool, the second thing I noted in the reports was that the chronological age at which interventions and/or strategies were applied was often directly linked to the likelihood of any initiative's success. According to a Dunedin paediatrician, for example:

> A child overweight at four has only a 40 percent chance of being normal weight as a teenager while an overweight teenager has an 80–90 percent likelihood of being an overweight adult.
>
> (Spratt 2006: 17)

It is difficult to locate the evidential source of these claims around specific ages and stages in a child's life where action must be taken and the point at which any effects will be nullified. It could be that developmental milestones derived from the discipline of developmental psychology are simply mapped on to youngsters in the context of obesity discourse in the way they are in relation to other issues (e.g. education and learning to walk), or there may be some biomedical evidence to support this capacity of experts to link a child's age to its chance of remediation. Whatever the case, these sources are not made available in the media reporting I analyzed.

Thirdly, one of the most alarming phenomenon emerging, as research findings from the escalating number of obesity studies are rolled out in

New Zealand's media, is the categorization of Maori and Pasifika peoples,[1] together with people of Asian heritage as the most problematic population sectors. The front-page headline in Wellington's *The Dominion* newspaper, Tuesday 14 November 2006 reads, 'Maori "facing extinction" from diabetes' followed by a lead in paragraph reporting that 'escalating rates of diabetes among indigenous cultures could make the Maori and Polynesian races "extinct" before the end of the century' (Torbitt 2006: 1). Drawing on the 'expert' testimony of an Australian Professor, we read that 'the rising number of diabetes victims among the world's indigenous communities would decimate entire cultures. Without urgent action there certainly is a real risk of a major wipeout of indigenous communities, if not total extinction, within this century' (Zimmet, quoted in Torbitt 2006: 1).

Whether or not these dire predictions have bases in empirical evidence is not the point here however. Rather, it is the persistent and widespread practice of the media linking type 2 diabetes with obesity and by association, with the dietary habits and exercise patterns of these indigenous communities with which I take issue. It is a not so complex conflation of ethnicity with class that marginalizes Maori and Pasifika peoples further than is already the case in obesity discourse. These groups are invariably and unsurprisingly positioned in the reporting and by the scientific community as more at risk than others. Their tendency to engage in cultural practices that involve celebrating rather than monitoring food, their avowed love affair with junk food and video parlours, their cultural practices that involve cooking up fatty mutton birds and consuming vast quantities of food at the peak of the food triangle (see Hokowhitu 2001) are represented as the 'truths' about Maori and ones that therefore place this group at more risk than anyone else in New Zealand. Cycles of poverty, disadvantage, violence and victimhood are phrases regularly used to describe the state of poor and/or Maori and Pasifika families (Bishop and Glynn 1999; Durie 1994) and it is little surprise that similar phrases are deployed in relation to these families and health. That is, the Maori obesity story is incorporated into a general disposition towards Maori that positions them as poor, criminals, truants, abusers and so on.

The kind of reportage alluded to above works to both constitute and regulate particular understandings of obesity risks, normality, morality and health. When this obesity story is aligned (as it is in most Western contexts) with neoliberal discourses emphasizing self-responsibility, free choice, autonomy, the knowledge economy, lifestyle and consumption (Larner 1998; Lauder and Hughes 1999), the allure of the obesity discourse and the normalizing practices it supports is readily understandable. The invocations to lose weight, manage one's health status, eat the 'right' foods, move one's body in ways conducive to the manufacture of an un-fat citizenry, and so on, hook into neo-liberal rationalities to produce what Bansel (2006) would refer to as a conceptual coupling. This is a coupling that urges parents and children in homes to enact technologies of the self (Foucault 1981) that will increase the likelihood of 'becoming' the healthy selves that *both* obesity discourse and neoliberal discourses inscribe as ideal. While there is considerable debate about the best *way/s* to actually get people to enact these lifestyle changes, central to the work of the agencies who profess to provide the tools is a commitment to the notion of a subject who can, with a little help choose to make the right choices amid the plethora of risky options that are out there (Burrows and Wright 2007).

With very small children (or indeed newborns) however, the route towards effecting change is less clear. As sociologists of childhood have pointed out (e.g. James and James 2004; Mayall 1996; Woodhouse 2004), children, have until relatively recently, in Western contexts, at least, been largely regarded as becomings rather than beings, as not yet fully formed, nor capable of making rational decisions in their own best interests. Thus, in the case of young children, parents and/or caregivers are often drawn into the obesity change project in very explicit ways, whether or not they would ordinarily choose to be so engaged (Burrows and Wright 2007). It is to some of the resources, tactics and strategies that parents are encouraged to embrace in their homes and families that I now turn.

PEDAGOGIZING PARENTS

As several curriculum writers have pointed out, pedagogy is a relational and complex practice, engaged in across multiple sites with the school being just one of these (Gore 1993; Lusted 1986). In the context of escalating concerns over childhood obesity, a startling array of parent-focused biopedagogies has arisen. The resources and techniques available to parents, whether they be public health, school-based, private agency or food industry generated are invariably focused on food, exercise, and/or sedentary behaviour and are available in an ever-expanding range of mediums, represented and designed in ways that match the ways parents and children currently access information (e.g. through the internet, doctors' surgeries, reality based television shows, public health campaigns, television advertising, popular culture and mail box flyers). What all of the resources and techniques are geared to do is convince parents that losing weight is a desirable family goal and to provide them with the requisite information and skills to achieve this. In biopedagogical terms, they operate at both the level of the individualized body and at the level of the species. That is, the instructions offered encourage individuals to divest themselves of personal body fat but *also* work as a form of state power, producing and distributing 'norms' related to body fat, weight, exercise and food consumption and offering forecasts, risk estimates and mortality rates related to obesity within the general population.

A review of Internet-based, television, and off-line resources for parents points to a proliferation of prescriptions related to the monitoring of television and other kinds of electronic media. The prescriptions range from screen-free time, to specifying TV allowances and physically removing televisions from children's bedrooms for the express reason of maximizing surveillance opportunities of children's activity. New Zealand's Ministry of Sport is launching a campaign that will 'challenge children and young people and their families to increase screen-free time from hours, to evenings, to days, to weekends' (SPARC 2006). As obesity commentator Bill Dietz puts it, 'parents must understand that supervising children's television use is as important as supervising their nutrition and schooling' (Levy 1999). Given the notable failure of 'just say no' tactics in other health spheres (e.g. drugs, smoking, sex and alcohol) it is challenging to understand how these strategies may actually work with children and young people, yet if these techniques fail, there are several alternative ones available to parents—techniques that actually make use of the so-called aberrant television and video games as rewards for good and healthful behaviour. For example, hooking up children's video game monitors to an exercycle and linking television viewing allowances to the number of steps recorded on personal pedometers.

Further, despite television being regarded as something families should watch less, there *is* a recognition that both television and radio *can* be used to 'reach' families en mass. New Zealand's *Mission-On*, for example, is planning funding of new programmes that focus on health food and physical activity choices, sponsoring segments on after-school shows to promote healthy eating and physical activity to children and featuring a group of lifestyle ambassadors whose brief is to show young people the route toward a healthy lifestyle. Similarly with web sites, New Zealand's Ministry of Sport and Recreation is developing 'interactive, dynamic and technologically savvy websites that . . ."push kid's buttons" to engage them in active learning (through fun) about healthy nutrition choices, physical activities, and related healthy lifestyles' (SPARC 2006). Sites are being designed for specific age brackets and offering features like 'pod casting, competitions, using "eye toys" and access to coaches, trainers and virtual buddies' (SPARC 2006). In the latter case, the virtual on-screen characters are in effect working as pedagogical puppets, conveying the 'instructions for life' authorized by New Zealand's Ministry of Health.

In regularizing mode, messages around children's physical activity for families are coming courtesy of a host of government initiatives including *Push Play*, *Mission On*, and the *Green Prescription*, together with a range of Ministry of Health resources distributed widely in schools, doctors' surgeries and community centres. For children, prescriptions for 'active living' are also broadcast via TV celebrities like SpongeBob SquarePants, the Teletubbies and other stars of children's popular culture. In disciplinary mode, websites like *Get Kids Active* (No Author 2006a) provide exhaustive lists of ways to get children moving and offer a range of products to help monitor children's maintenance of physical activity regimes. In school programmes, children at all levels are encouraged as part of their health and physical education curriculum to fill in daily diaries detailing what they've eaten, how much activity they've done and how they feel about it. Family fat camps and special programmes for at risk kids involving the whole family are also emerging courtesy of New Zealand's *Active Families* network (SPARC 2007). These programmes involve an intensive and ongoing level of monitoring of children's weight, girth and activity levels with follow up advice and support offered to families who really want to help their children lose weight. I would suggest that this is an intense level of surveillance of self and by others that is at work here.

Furthermore, medical advice regarding weight surveillance throughout infancy to childhood is regularly recited in both popular media and resources designed for parents. For example, according to Dr Nicolas Stettler, an American paediatrician, whose study is repeatedly quoted in newspaper reports, 'early infancy seems to be a critical period for the establishment of obesity. Babies double their birth weight during the first four to six months, so this may be a period for the establishment of weight regulation' (http://www.rsnz.org/news/news_item.php?view=10993, posted on 05/02/02 Accessed on 19 September 06). While not all media reports and resources encourage the weighing of children, many do promote a visual monitoring of the shape and weight of children within families, together with the notion that considerable effort will be required to change one's weight and shape in pursuit of 'health'. The ways in which such 'expert' knowledge can be taken up and disseminated via school contexts, is exemplified in a New Zealand school newsletter where the principal instructs parents in the following way: '[i]f an overweight child is ready to put the effort into getting healthier, she/he will need help . . . Discuss with the child the truth that losing weight and getting in better shape takes effort. Talk to them about how weight and body shape run in families' (Jenkins 2006: 1).

It is with food that mothers, in particular, as presumed keepers of the kitchen are encouraged to be especially vigilant about not only what their children consume within the home but outside it as well (Murphy, Parker and Phipps 2001). In New Zealand, a burgeoning market for family health cookbooks has emerged with agencies like the New Zealand Dietetics Association taking up a monitoring role in relation to the quality of each new release. Adult healthy food magazines feature hot tips on how to trick children into consuming 'healthy' foods, while internet family health sites offer games like *Panic Picnic* that children can play with or without their parents. The winners are those who refrain from adding ice creams or biscuits to their picnic basket. As is the case with physical exercise, the quantities and quality of the food ingested is prescribed in clear, if conflicting ways across the range of resources parents have access to. These practices work to constitute norms around what constitutes a 'good' diet, divide food into good and bad groups and invite simplistic and I would add boring prescriptions for how one should eat one's way through life. Further the capacity of parents to enact dietary recommendations serves up yet another opportunity for comparison, judgement and evaluation of parents' capacity to care in the right way. For example, the results of lunch-box checks happening in schools across New Zealand (and Canada and Australia) serve as visible indicators of the vigilance (or not) of parents—the lunch-box functioning, in effect, as a sign of parental care.

Together with the surveillant, monitoring, normalizing and role modelling techniques alluded to above, parental *participation* in the lives and education of children also emerges as a pivotal disciplinary technique for fostering children's capacity to adopt obesity reduction practices. The Internet parenting sites, books and school-based resources themselves are replete with advice that foregrounds the importance of parents joining in children's activities. This brings the child and parent into a pedagogical relation allowing further surveillance by parents of children and of course, requiring of parents a great deal of time and energy (something that professionals lament low socio-economic group parents aren't always willing to give).

THE EFFECTS

The kinds of instructions I have discussed thus far are not necessarily in themselves aberrant. Rather, what is troublesome is the way a parent's capacity to manage these imperatives—in both in media reportage and so-called scientific accounts of obesity—is mapped onto notions of what constitutes a good parent per se. That is, within obesity discourse, a failure to role model healthy citizenship and a failure to deliver on the recommended strategies for producing un-fat children effectively wipes out any other contribution to the upbringing of a well child that parent/s may have made.

The potential effects of failing to give children a good start on parents' sense of their capacity to raise their children is powerfully demonstrated on New Zealand's new reality television series *Honey We're Killing the Kids*—a show that regularly reduces parents (predominantly mothers) to tears as it points out parental negligence and its likely effects on the children they profess to care for. The central premise of the show is that if parents don't do something now they are in fact contributing to the death of their children. In October 2006 a Pasifika family worried about the bulging tummy of their 9 year-old were taken under the reality show's wing. Instructions on menu planning together with digitally enhanced projections of what little Henry would look like unless the parents (read mother) changed his diet assisted this family to make 'grocery shopping and exercise a family affair' (Spratt 2006: 20). As reported in the *New Zealand Listener* during this show, 'Iona (the mum) learnt that she was using too much fat in her cooking and too much junk food in the kids' lunchboxes. She still cries when she talks about the photo the show mocked up of what Henry would look like if he didn't change his lifestyle. As she exclaimed, "It wasn't our Henry, it was horrible. We were killing him"' (Spratt 2006: 20). This message is clear, Henry is at risk, the mother is responsible, and changes will require the entire family to change their lifestyles.

What is thought provoking about the aforementioned show and the raft of family focused resources emerging to address obesity in childhood, is the invocation to parents to engage the whole family in weight managing and watching strategies and the implication that doing so will in itself build stronger and happier families. By the end of the show, the aforementioned family were sitting down to eat together, being nicer to each other and the grand finale was a scene where they were all rewarded for their efforts by a family bungy jump experience. The mother looked terrified, but the event was symbolic of a functioning family, who can have fun together, encourage each other, and perform as a good neoliberal family should. As Bansel (2006) suggests, the practices and dispositions a so-called neoliberal family embraces are inevitably premised on westerncentric and middle-class values yet unproblematically portrayed as an 'ideal' applicable to all.

In a sense, it is an intensification of the well-worn message 'a family who plays together stays together'. New Zealand's Ministry of Sport draws explicitly on this motto in the latest of their *Push Play* campaigns—a nationwide competition to gauge which families (and by association) communities can be the most active in a given period of time. In December 2006 families were invited to display a green *Get It Up* balloon outside their homes to show others that they were a *Push Play* household. The competition involves recording amounts of physical activity engaged in each day on a score sheet provided by the Ministry of Sport and Recreation. This is a very public display of one's adherence (or not) to what government regards as crucial self-disciplinary practices. How families come to understand their worth is symbolized by the practices they enact (or don't) in their homes, in their own time, in the private sphere.

What these, and other practices like it do, is admonish everyone in a family (or community) to pull their weight—not to do so, is to jeopardize the entire family's success—to continue to eat bad foods lie on the couch and watch the telly while some family members are trying to make a change is regarded as a lack of support. In *Fighting Fat*—yet another fat busting reality show—participants are viewed struggling to maintain their dietary and exercise regimes in families that don't share their desire to lose weight and refuse to change their own practices to match those of the fat fighter.

> Our biggest fat fighter Craig is about to go on a road trip. About 60 kms into the journey it's as per the family tradition the 2.5-hour drive is littered with pit stops a long the way . . . he needs to be strong but it's not going to be easy. I do feel guilty eating it cos dad can't (daughter). But Craig has an empty stomach and a clean conscience.
>
> (TVNZ 2006)

The 'good' family responds in the way this Teawamutu family who themselves appeared on *Honey We're Killing the Kids* does:

As a family, we wanted to show other families that healthy eating, and more importantly a healthy lifestyle, can be achieved, and that we owe it to our children to give them the knowledge so that we can be secure in knowing that they will make wise choices that benefit their lives, now and in the future.

(No Author 2006b)

This kind of family-to-family snowball effect, I suggest, exemplifies how biopedagogical practices are meant to work.

Each of the biopedagogies examined thus far work not only at the level of the material body (to shape, tone and work bodies to fit a healthy 'norm') but also to produce and reproduce subjects (i.e. parents and children) within families, their practices and beliefs and their relationships with each other. Parental guilt and shame are powerful motivators for the families who feature on programmes like *Honey We're Killing the Kids*. The programme provides not only opportunities for the public to watch parents' recognition of themselves as abject (Kristeva 1982), but also ready access to the emotions provoked when parents 'understand' the debilitating effects their family lifestyle is having on their offspring. In a sense, the programme invites us all to evaluate the way we 'do' family, to surveille our family members, manage their behaviours and to assess ourselves and our families against the aberrant ones the programme confronts us with.

The phenomenon of watching other people who themselves are being watched can be regarded as an extraordinary addition to the tactics of governance and particularly to neoliberal styles of governance. When techniques of categorization, normalization and family surveillance are beamed into thousands of homes, the boundaries between institutionalized pedagogy (e.g. what goes on in schools) and the kinds of educative practices that go on in homes are blurred. The family, in a sense becomes an additional biopedagogical arm that encourages us to 'participate in the governance of our own bodies and lives, and in the bodies and lives of others' (Bansel 2006: 3). It is, in effect, another step en route to what Bernstein (1996: 366) terms a 'totally pedagogised society'.

Bordo (1992), Shilling (1993), Tinning (1985) and others have eloquently written about the ways social capital is read off the body in contemporary times, and rather than reiterate their arguments here, I want to suggest that in the context of obesity discourse, these tendencies are influencing not only how individuals regard themselves and others but also, how families are constituted and regarded as 'functional' and 'good'. The normative family as construed in programmes like *Honey We're Killing the Kids* and in *Push Play* initiatives and 'healthy food' magazines is the same one that health product media advertisers want consumers to desire—that is, a good neoliberal family embracing market choice, consumerism, self autonomy and lifestyle aspirations (e.g. bungy jumping) that are reflective of health *and* wealth. Being outwardly healthy, something generally equated with not being fat, is not just part of the neoliberal family package, but, I would argue, is in and of itself an outward marker of having become a fine neoliberal family. As numerous policy studies analysts have explained, some families (and indeed, I would contend *most* families) simply don't and won't fit this ideal and in New Zealand at least, it is non-European, particularly Maori, Pasifika peoples and latterly families of Asian descent (Indian in particular) who are disproportionately represented across all indices as failing to create and nurture the 'good' family.

Further, orthodox assumptions about links between social-class positioning and behaviour are only very thinly veiled in the technologies advanced. The New Zealand government is currently discussing the merits of cutting tax on fruit as an incentive to encourage healthy eating. A New Zealand Ministry of Sport and Recreation official had this to say about the proposed tax cuts on fruit: '[t]he people who already eat well will be smiling . . . while those who choose a $1 pie and Coke because it's cheaper than healthy food are the same people who will be renting DVDs, smoking and buying Lotto tickets. It's all about priorities' (cited in Spratt 2006: 18). The invocation of choice as a rational matter is clear here. Poor people, on this account, will not make the right choices even when they are offered to them on a plate (like the tax free fruit scheme). The reasons for this apparent failure to do the right thing are variously attributed in popular media and research reports (e.g. Fight the Obesity Epidemic 2008; Tagata Pasifika 2007; Taylor 2007; Torbitt 2006) to poor education, a culturally induced reticence to engage with mainstream discourse, and a mistaken belief that they are alright as they are.

CONCLUSION

The pedagogization of families I have attempted to describe above entails a fascinating juxtaposition of neoliberalist discourses with those associated by some with the 'nanny-state' (see Gard in this book)—the former emphasizing self-governing accountable individuals who make rational and autonomous choices about their health regardless of context—and the latter, emphasizing the vulnerability of children and the different realities of families' lives that render state intervention and assistance crucial, particularly in the lives of indigenous and minority groups and those regarded as working-class. So-called 'nanny-state' policies would normally be vociferously attacked by New Zealand's conservative opposition government yet with obesity there is not even a murmur of dissent. As Gard (2007) points out, there is something about the couplet of 'child' and 'obesity' and, I would argue, the couplet of obesity and ethnicity that makes it palatable to dissolve private/public barriers and intervene in the micropractices of families' lives.

Further, the moral dimensions of neoliberal rationalities that arise in obesity discourse are of particular concern. The positioning of families who do not engage with the tools provided them in positive ways as negligent is disturbing. Postcolonial scholars in NZ like Brendan Hokowhitu provide commentary on how Maori families regard food and physical activity that yields insights about why Maori disproportionately tend to resist the kinds of biopedagogical advances Pakeha (non-Maori) advance upon them. He draws on the testimony of pakeke (esteemed Maori physical educators) to show that concepts like fitness, fatness, and even health itself have distinct meanings (or none at all in the case of fitness) within Maori culture, meanings that bear little relation to the kind enunciated in the plethora of government and private agency sponsored initiatives geared towards reducing fat in these populations. The failure to engage with diverse and potentially productive ways of regarding these ideas is thought-provoking. Indeed, in a climate where diversity is claimed to be valued everywhere from consumer culture to government policy, popular culture and education, it seems extraordinary that such a monocultural vision of the 'ideal' body can gain so much prominence and that the notion of what constitutes a good and healthful family can be so narrowly defined. The slogans gracing New Zealand television screens currently courtesy of *Mission-On* are 'we're all in this together' and 'this is how "we" do it', yet the 'we' invoked is barely recognizable to large chunks of the nation. Perhaps, we can as Davies and Bansel (2006: 6) suggest, look not so much to the individual or family as being at the heart of these practices but rather to the 'institutional regimes and practices through which we are managed, and hold those institutions responsible and accountable for the lives of the subjects they govern?'

NOTES

1. In the context of New Zealand, Pasifika refers to the different ethnicities that collectively comprise the Pacific Island communities of New Zealand. Maori refers to the indigenous peoples of Aotearoa/New Zealand.

REFERENCES

Archard, D. (1993) *Children: Rights and Childhood*, London: Routledge.
Aries, P. (1962) *Centuries of Childhood: A Social History of Family Life*, London: Jonathan Cape.
Bansel, P. (2006) 'Subjects of choice', a paper presented at *Tracing Neo-liberalism Across Multiple Sites* symposium, University Of Otago, Dunedin, 4 December.
Bernstein, B. (1996) *Pedagogy, Symbolic Control and Identity: Theory Research and Critique*, London: Taylor and Francis.
Bird, L. (1994) 'Creating the Capable Body: Discourses About Ability and Effort in Primary and Secondary School Subjects', in B. Mayall (ed.) *Children's Childhoods: Observed and Experienced*, London: The Falmer Press.
Bishop, R. and Glynn, T. (1999) *Culture Counts*, Palmerston North: Dunmore.

Bordo, S. (1992) 'The Body and the Reproduction of Femininity: A Feminist Appropriation of Foucault', in A.M. Jaggar and S.R. Bordo (eds) *Gender/Body/ Knowledge*, New Brunswick: Rutgers University Press.

Burman, E. (1991) *Power, Gender and Developmental Psychology*, London: Routledge.

Burrows, L. and Wright, J. (2007) 'Prescribing practices: Shaping healthy children in schools', *International Journal of Children's Rights*, 15: 83–98.

Campos, P. (2004) *The Obesity Myth: Why America's Obsession with Weight is Hazardous to Your Health*, United States: Gotham Books.

Campos, P., Saguy, A., Ernsberger, P., Oliver, E. and Gaesser, G. (2006) 'The epidemiology of overweight and obesity: public health crisis or moral panic?', *International Journal of Epidemiology*, 35(1): 55–60.

Clark, H. (2006) *Mission-On: HealthyLlifestyles for Young Kiwis*: retrieved 24 July 2008, from http://www.beehive.govt.nz/ViewDocument.aspx? DocumentID=27181>

Davies, B. and Bansel, P. (2006) 'The time of their lives? Academic workers in neo-liberal time(s)' paper presented at *Tracing Neo-liberalism Across Multiple Sites* symposium, University Of Otago, Dunedin, 4 December.

Dreyfus, H.L. and Rabinow, P. (1982) *Michel Foucault: Beyond Structuralism and Hermeneutics*, London: Haverster Wheatsheaf.

Durie, M. (1994) *Whaiora: Maori Health Development*, Auckland: Oxford University Press.

Fight the Obesity Epidemic (2008) *Obesity: The Facts*: retrieved 2 January 2008, from http://www.foe.org.nz/facts3.html

Foucault, M. (1977) *Discipline and Punish: The Birth of the Prison*, London: Penguin.

Foucault, M. (1981) *The History of Sexuality: An Introduction*, Hammondsworth: Penguin.

Foucault, M. (1991) 'Bio-power: Right of Death and Power Over Life', in P. Rainbow (ed.) *The Foucault Reader*, London: Penguin.

Foucault, M. (2003) *Society Must be Defended: Lectures at the College de France 1975–76*, New York: Picador.

Gard, M. and Wright, J. (2005) *The Obesity Epidemic: Science, Morality and Ideology*, London: Routledge.

Gore, J. (1993) *The Struggle for Pedagogies: Critical and Feminist Discourses as Regimes of Truth*, New York: Routledge.

Hokowhitu, B. (2001) *Te mana Maori—Te tatari i nga korero parau*, unpublished thesis, University of Otago, Dunedin.

James, A. and James, A.L. (2004) *Constructing Childhood: Theory, Policy and Social Practice*, New York: Palgrave/MacMillan.

Jenkins, T. (2006) 'Helping an overweight child', *East Otago High School Newsletter Week 3 Term Four*, 27 October: 1.

Kristeva, J. (1982) *Powers of Horror: An Essay on Abjection*, trans. Leon Roudiez, New York: Columbia University Press.

Larner, W. (1998) 'Sociologies of neo-liberalism: Theorising the "New Zealand experiment"', *Sites*, 36: 5–21.

Lauder, H. and Hughes, D. (1999) *Trading in Futures: Why Markets in Education Don't Work*, Buckingham: Open University Press.

Levy, D. (1999) *TV Replacing Play, Family Time for Kiwi Kids*, posted 12 October: retrieved 19 September 2006, from http://www.rsnz.org/news/news_item. php?view=158

Lusted, D. (1986) 'Why pedagogy', *Screen*, 27(5): 2–15.

Mayall, B. (1996) *Children, Health and the Social Order*, Buckingham: Open University Press.

Mayall, B. (1998) 'Towards a sociology of child health', *Sociology of Health Illness*, 20: 269–88.

Murphy, E., Parker, S. and Phipps, C. (2001) 'Motherhood, Morality, and Infant Feeding', in J. Germov and L. Williams (eds) *A Sociology of Food and Nutrition: The Social Appetite*, Victoria: Oxford University Press.

No Author (2006a) *Get Kids Active*: retrieved 19 November 2006, from http://www.getkidsactive.com

No Author (2006b) *Te Awamutu Online*: retrieved 25 November 2006, from www.teawamutu.co.nz

Reuters (2002) *Studies Show Health Dangers of Overfeeding Infants*, posted 5 February: retrieved 19 September 2006, from http://www.rsnz.org/news/news_item.php?view=10993

Shilling, C. (1993) *The Body and Social Theory*, London: Sage.

Sport and Recreation New Zealand (SPARC) (2006) *Mission-On Fact Sheet*: retrieved 20 November 2006, from http://www.sparc.org.nz/filedownload?id=d3effde9–7415–44e7-a357–87380992a776

Sport and Recreation New Zealand (SPARC) (2007) *No Exceptions: Strategy and Implementation Plan 2005—2009*: retrieved 20 January 2007, from http://www.sparc.org.nz/filedownload?id=70dc299d-9d7a-42f8-b5cf-ede073c60da3

Spratt, A. (2006) 'The big picture', *New Zealand Listener*, 18–24 November: 14–20.

Tagata Pasifika (2007) *Child Obesity in New Zealand Study*: retrieved 2 January 2008, from http://www.tnz.co.nz/view/page/410965/1448684

Taylor, R. (2007) 'What's hot and what's not', keynote address presented at *New Zealand Health Teachers' Association Conference: 'Our Health, Our Children, Our Future'*, Dunedin, 30 June–3 July.

Tinning, R. (1985) 'Physical education and the cult of slenderness: a critique', *ACHPER National Journal*, 107: 10–14.

Torbitt, T. (2006) 'Diabetes could "wipe out" Maori by end of century', *The Dominion*, 14 November: 1.

TVNZ (2006) *One Shows A to Z: Fighting Fat* : retrieved 20 December 2006, from http://tvnz.co.nz/view/page/410965/945999

Walkerdine, V. (1984) 'Developmental Psychology and the Child-Centred Pedagogy: The Insertion of Piaget Into Early Education', in W. Henriques, C. Hollway, C. Urin, C. Venn and V. Walkerdine (eds) *Changing the Subject: Psychology, Social Regulation and Subjectivity*, London: Methuen.

Woodhouse, B. (2004) 'Re-visioning Rights for Children', in P. Pufall and R. Unsworth (eds) *Rethinking Childhood*, New Jersey: Rutgers University Press.

Wyn, J. and White, R. (1997) *Rethinking Youth*, St Leonards: Allen and Unwin.

10 Canadian Youth's Discursive Constructions of Health in the Context of Obesity Discourse

Geneviève Rail

OBESITY DISCOURSE

Few will have escaped the avalanche of scientific and public comments about obesity in the last few years. Escalating concerns over an 'obesity epidemic' have been fuelled by the dramatic increase of epidemiological, physiological and medical literature on obesity (see an overview in Gard and Wright 2005) and its recuperation by the media, educational institutions, health and fitness practitioners, and public health officials. This crisis is said to afflict an increasing number of countries in the world and threatens a global health catastrophe (WHO 2000). The World Health Organization has even declared obesity a 'disease' (WHO 2006).

More recently, obesity research has been critiqued from a number of angles. Both social scientists and biomedical researchers have challenged the use of the term 'epidemic' (Campos, Saguy, Ernsberger, Oliver and Gaesser 2006; Gard 2004), the notion of obesity as a disease (Gaesser 2003; Oliver 2006), the burden of disease due to obesity (Gaesser and Blair 2002, Mark 2005), the attribution of deaths to obesity (Farrell, Braun, Barlow, Cheng and Blair 2002; Flegal, Graubard, Williamson and Gail 2005) and the identification of obesity as a public health priority (Campos et al. 2006; Gard and Wright 2005). These authors and others have also noted contradictions regarding obesity's measurement, causes, solutions and interventions (Herrick 2007; Holm 2007; Komesaroff and Thomas 2007). Finally, a number of scholars, including contributors to this book, have questioned the medicalization of obese individuals as well as those 'at-risk' for obesity (Murray 2007 and 2008; Oliver 2006).

While these critical debates raise significant questions, they have taken place away from the public, and media stories feeding anxieties over obesity have continued to flourish (Saguy and Almeling 2007). Researchers have documented the explosion of scientific and media reports on obesity in the United States (Campos 2004; Oliver 2005), Australia (Gard and Wright 2005), and England (Evans et al. 2004; Evans, Rich and Davies 2005). These authors have invariably recognized a dominant 'obesity discourse'. This discourse offers a mechanistic view of the body and focuses on the assumed relationship between inactivity, poor diet, obesity and health. In the same breath, it presents obesity in moral and economic terms: obese and 'at-risk' bodies are constructed as lazy and expensive bodies that should be submitted to expert investigation (Groskopf 2005). Against suggestions that the food industry, the car culture, consumer society and other socio-cultural factors play a role in the development of an 'obesogenic environment' (Boehmer, Lovegreen, Haire-Joshu and Brownson 2006; Lang and Rayner 2007; Nestle 2002), short, uncomplicated and people-centred explanations that are well suited for the media dominate in obesity discourse, often excluding or marginalizing important considerations around the influence of social structure.

The dominant obesity discourse has generated new forms of normalizing practices to reduce obesity and to protect everyone from the 'risks' of obesity (see more on this in Chapter 1, this volume). Such practices place individuals under constant surveillance and press them towards monitoring themselves. They draw upon a neo-liberal notion of individualism that positions individuals as primarily responsible for changing their lifestyle in relation to exercise and diet (Campos 2004). Within obesity discourse, both overweight and obesity are represented as a failure to care for one's self while the thin body is given recognition as reflecting control, virtue and goodness (Evans, Rich and Davies 2004; Rich and Evans 2005). Obesity discourse thus incites disciplinary processes of pathologization of fat and ascription of deviance (Murray 2007, and Chapter 6 in this book). In his work on the 'McDonaldization' of overweight bodies, Monaghan (2007) has written about some of the principles (e.g. calculability, efficiency, predictability and technological control) that are being harnessed for the public and private fight against fat.

Researchers in a number of countries have recently reported on the ways disciplinary practices have been encouraged across a range of cultural practices including popular media (Burrows and Wright 2004), new technologies (Miah and Rich 2006), health organizations (Groskopf 2005) and schools (Gallagher and Fusco 2006; Ikeda, Amy, Ernsberger, Gaesser, Berg, Clark, Parham and Peters 2005; Vertinsky 2004). Although we are only starting to interrogate the situation in Canada, there is some evidence (e.g. MacNeill and Rail 2007) regarding the plethora of school, health promotion, and public health programs that are targeting youth obesity and deploying a whole range of disciplinary practices to curtail it.

DISCURSIVE EFFECTS

While obesity research and debates have received much scholarly attention, there has been minimal discussion on the material and embodied effects of obesity discourse and biopedagogies. Some psychological studies have suggested that media images contribute to body dissatisfaction, particularly among young women (see an overview in Grogan 1999).

Researchers working with anorexic young women (e.g. Rich and Evans 2005) have also suggested that obesity discourse could lead to forms of size discrimination and oppression that propel some women toward ill-health via disordered relationships with food, exercise and the body. Researchers working with overweight and 'obese' individuals (e.g. Annis, Cash and Hrabosky 2007; Friedman, Reichmann, Costanzo, Zelli, Ashmore and Musante 2005) have reported body dissatisfaction, distress, weight preoccupation, increased binge eating, lower self-esteem, fewer social networks, less social capital, and less satisfaction with life. But the way obesity discourse is taken up by ordinary youth (with a variety of weights and shapes) has only recently been touched upon (e.g. Wright, O'Flynn, and Macdonald 2006).

A number of feminist theorists have directed their attention to the ways in which women negotiate socio-cultural ideals of femininity associated with the body (e.g. Bartky 1990; Bordo 1993; Orbach 1988). Feminist, queer and disability theorists have also addressed the social constructions of fatness and challenged the power relations and oppressive practices associated with such constructions (e.g. Braziel and Lebesco 2001; Butler 1990; Garland-Thomson 2005; Grosz 1994). In sum, feminist scholars have presented *theoretical* writings on weight and obesity and these lead to a number of critical questions that have rarely been answered empirically. For instance, how do individuals negotiate the dominant discourse of obesity? What effect does this discourse have on individuals' conceptualization of the body and health or on bodily practices? In the paragraphs that follow, I present a modest attempt to start answering these questions by looking at the connections between obesity discourse and youth's discursive constructions of health. This examination is part of a larger collaborative investigation of Canadian youth's constructions of health and fitness (Rail, Beausoleil, MacNeill, Burrows and Wright 2003–7, project funded by the Social Sciences and Humanities Research Council of Canada).

EXPLORING THE EFFECTS OF OBESITY DISCOURSE: THEORETICAL AND METHODOLOGICAL CONSIDERATIONS

In this chapter, I use a poststructuralist perspective (Rail 2002; Weedon 1997; Wright 2001) to explore the discursive effects of the dominant obesity discourse. This framework allows for an understanding of *subjectivity* as decentred and being made possible and constituted through the already gendered, heterosexualized and racialized discourses to which one has access; as a subject, one is *interpellated* or 'hailed' (Butler 1997) by various subject positions. The poststructuralist framework is underpinned by a number of other key concepts. My use of the term *construction* reflects the poststructuralist notion that reality is made and not found. Young people construct 'reality' through language and cultural practices. Following Foucault (1973), I see *discourses* as 'regimes of truth' that specify what can be said or done at particular times and places, and that sustain specific relations of power (Rail and Harvey 1995). This generates questions about how *power* is exercised in the construction of *knowledge* about obesity and health, and about what kinds of knowledge are legitimized. I see *identity* as dynamic and multiple. Identity is negotiated in relation to various sets of meanings and practices that youth draw on as they participate in the bodily and wider culture and come to understand who they are (George and Rail 2006). In this sense, identity involves a notion of *performativity* (Butler 1990 and 1997): a re-experiencing of meanings associated with gender, sexuality, dis/ability, race, ethnicity, etc., that are already socially established. This perspective also draws from writings (e.g., Bhabha 1994; Minh-Ha 1995; Spivak 1995) that allow for a conceptualisation of experiences in a *postcolonial* way in the sense that they avoid the pitfalls of abstraction and generalization.

In line with the above theoretical considerations, the study presented in this chapter relied on a poststructuralist discourse analysis method (Lupton 1992; Rail 2002; Weedon 1997; Wright 1995) to investigate how young people's narratives are connected to a wider social and cultural context infused with discourses about health, obesity, and the body. Such narratives were gathered through one-on-one conversations and small group discussions with young Canadians from the Ottawa and Toronto areas. The conversation and discussion guides were developed both in French and English. Small group discussions were conducted with 13–15 years old students from Grade 9 physical education classes in French- and English-language schools. In addition, one-on-one conversations or small group discussions were organized with English-speaking youth (all 13–16 years old except for a few women in their late teens and early twenties) coming from the Korean-Canadian, the South-Asian-Canadian, the Portuguese-Canadian and the Somali-Canadian communities. Adolescents with a mobility impairment also took part in conversations. Recruitment and participation conditions (e.g. participant, school, community and parental consents) were laid out as required in the University of Ottawa ethical guidelines. The purposive sample (a total of 75 young men and 69 young women) allowed for the inclusion of young people from a range of socio-cultural locations.

Conversations and discussions were audio-taped, transcribed (using the pseudonyms included here), and then submitted successively to thematic and poststructuralist analyses. The analyses focused on how participants discursively construct health, how they—as subjects—position and construct themselves within dominant or resistant discourses, on the role obesity discourse plays in such constructions, and on the ways in which meanings about health are constructed in specific socio-cultural circumstances. The results of the analyses are presented in the next section.

Table 10.1   Young Canadians' Discursive Constructions of Health

Health Is	# of Mentions
Being physically active	581
Eating well	486
Being not too fat, looking good, being not too skinny	445
Having other physical qualities	230
Avoiding bad habits	193
Having personal qualities	184
Being happy, feeling good	138
Not being sick	72
Having a healthy environment, good friends	38

N = 144 participants

DISCURSIVE CONSTRUCTIONS OF HEALTH

Virtually all of the young people in this study were very familiar with the dominant discourses on the body and health. These discourses found their way into their constructions of health as they emerged from their narratives. As is shown in Table 10.1, nine 'themes' characterized such constructions of health.

An examination of the above themes leads to a number of conclusions. First and most importantly, we can say that the participants emphasized three themes related to the dominant obesity discourse: 'being physically active', 'eating well', and 'being not too fat'. Not only were these themes overwhelming in the participants' narratives, but the way in which they were connected to each other convincingly reflected the obesity discourse's mechanistic conceptualisation of the body: avoiding obesity (being not too fat) is simply a question of caloric intake (eating well) and output (being physically active). Second, health was mostly constructed in bodily terms and was either associated with things that are done to the body (e.g. being physically active, eating well, avoiding bad habits) or that are associated with the body (e.g. being neither too fat nor too skinny, having physical qualities, not being sick). Much less frequently, participants described health in non-corporeal terms such as 'feeling good' and 'having personal qualities'. Third, despite the omnipresence of negative messages about smoking, unprotected sex, drugs or alcohol in Canadian public health messages targeting youth, it is interesting to find out that avoiding such 'bad habits' was not so present in the constructions of health. This seems to be a good example of government and school messages being like droplets in the ocean of dominant cultural discourses about the body (i.e. the importance of not being fat and of looking good). Fourth and last, the participants' constructions of health are such that they integrate the discourse of individual responsibility for health: health is something that they are (e.g. thin, confident, positive, fit, not sick), that they do (e.g. physical activity, eating well, avoiding bad habits) or that they feel (e.g. feeling good). Such integration is quite dramatic when we know that the most important determinants of health in Canada (e.g. socio-economic status, education, employment, physical and social environment) reside at the macro-level and that micro-level determinants (lifestyle, genes) have only a modest impact on population health (Raphael 2003; Wilkinson and Marmot 1998).

OBESITY DISCOURSE AND THE IMPORTANCE OF 'NOT BEING LAZY'

The most significant element in the participants' constructions of health was 'being physically active'. The latter meant participating in organized or unorganized physical activities, exercises, and sports. Within their narratives on physical activity, participants emphasized the regularity of involvement and attributed positive personal qualities to people who take part in regular physical activity. Tommy, Kimberly and Maria (Korean-Canadian adolescents) stated that healthy people keep an active lifestyle:

> **Tommy:** He [Tommy's friend with whom he plays basketball] works out, so he is masculine. He plays a lot of sports, too. So, he is healthy.
> **Kimberly:** Being healthy means being basically active whatever you do.
> **Maria:** They [unhealthy people] are mostly overweight, [they] don't really participate in [physical education] classes [like] healthier people, and probably in the gym, they always run slower on running [machines].

In addition to 'being physically active', participants used expressions such as 'not being lazy', 'not being a couch potato' and talked about other markers of sedentary lifestyles like watching TV and being in front of a computer. The obesity discourse was clearly re-articulated by most participants. The notion of individual responsibility for one's health translated into the notion of self-responsibility for one's lifestyle and the idea that lazy people have lazy lifestyles and are not so healthy. The young people used many moral terms to qualify the 'lazy' individuals but qualifiers used to describe others were not applied to themselves. In line with this, most participants considered themselves 'healthy' despite the fact that few reported being involved in regular sport, exercise or fitness activities.

Whatever their physical and 'health' practices, the young people in the study were very aware of health messages coming from school and community programs. They could easily re-articulate messages linking physical activity to health. That being said, they associated health practices with accessible but 'boring' everyday activities (e.g. moving, being physically active, eating well). As for fitness, it was associated with performance, perseverance, athletic achievement and uncomfortable physical exertion, in other words, activities that are seen as difficult, not enjoyable, and seldom part of their every day life since they required specialized knowledge, time, money and access to 'the best place to do it'.

OBESITY DISCOURSE AND THE
IMPORTANCE OF 'NOT BEING FAT'

The participants' constructions of health involved a crucial link to bodily shape. For all of them, health meant having a particular body shape and weight and, more specifically, being not too fat, overweight or obese, and being thin or skinny. Not surprisingly, given the dominant discourse linking obesity to ill-health, 'fat' individuals were readily considered as unhealthy and 'slim', 'regular' or 'not too fat' people (categories in which most of them included themselves) tended to be stereotyped as healthy, as is evident in Score's (Korean-Canadian young man) narrative:

> [I'm healthy because I'm not fat and] I'm trying not to get fat or anything. Like, I don't really look at my weight as scare-wise, like, fat or anything. I just sort of check myself in the mirror and see if my stomach is bulging out, something like that [demonstrating and laughing]. You know you can't have that kind of thing. That's not a good sign. You know, we all want healthy bodies and we all want to be shaped.

The above quote illustrates how elements of the obesity discourse were recycled as universal truths ('we all want . . . and we all want to be') that speak not only to self-regulation but the regulation of others.

A majority of participants also constructed health as 'not being too skinny'. For young men, being too skinny generally meant not having sufficient muscles and for young women, it was associated with anorexia and ill-health. Most male and female participants regarded themselves as being and appearing 'healthy' even if they did not all appreciate their own bodily appearance. As is demonstrated in the following discussion among high-school students, some participants were also quick to associate certain bodies with ill-health:

> **Maxwell:** [Unhealthy people are] fat people, skinny people, ugly-looking people.
>
> **Charlie:** People with disabilities, people with Down's syndrome or something like that.
>
> **Josianne:** So you judge them by their appearance?
>
> **Charlie:** Physical, it's mostly physical appearance cause if you don't go talk to them, you don't know. If it's a complete stranger, then you judge them by appearance.

A number of participants offered resistance to the dominant (ableist) discourse that equates health to a particular physical appearance. Like Charlie, a few of them suggested that you could not tell if someone is healthy just by looking at them. This was particularly the case for young people with a mobility impairment. Jim, for instance, explained that his experience of playing wheelchair basketball had shown him a few things:

> I can't describe it [a healthy body]. It's different for everybody. Everybody is healthy in their own way, it doesn't matter what they look like . . . Like, I know people who are half a person [laughs], only have half a body but they are still in good shape and they are still healthy people.

In contrast to young people with a mobility impairment, a majority of the participants across all other socio-cultural locations constructed health in terms of having a 'normal' body and this normality seemed to be perceived differently by males and females. In general, young men alluded to the normal body as not fat, muscular and well shaped. For young women, being slim and toned corresponded to a female's 'proper' body shape. The participants' gendered view of the body was most evident in their consideration of muscles. For instance, when asked if women should have muscles, Abigail (high-school student) stated:

> **Abigail:** Yeah, but not too much.
> **Josianne:** Why not?
> **Abigail:** That would be just too much; she would look like she's on drugs or something.
> **Josianne:** Could you describe to me what a healthy guy would look like?
> **Abigail:** He would have a lot of muscles because guys have muscles and less body fat.

While female participants considered big muscles unattractive for women, male participants read muscularity as a sign of masculinity and male health. Youth narratives were highly gendered however it seemed as though the concern was more about 'looking good' or 'not being fat' than about 'being healthy'. As an example, when asked if he cared about his health, Matt (high school student) answered: '[y]eah, I care a little bit right now. I know I'm gonna care a lot more when I'm older, but right now, I think I'm OK. I'm not too concerned about it, unless I get too fat'. For most participants, health seemed to be something they already had whereas 'not being fat' and 'looking good' seemed to be things on which they needed to work. This is well illustrated in the following excerpt:

Healthy to me means, um, taking care of your body, like maintaining a decent weight, looking presentable, you know, like being healthy and fit. I think if you work on your body, you'll look good, feel good and you'll also be healthy.

(Cindy, young South-Asian Canadian woman)

More so than for the young men, the young women in the study reported subjecting themselves to bodily disciplines to meet the requirements of conventional femininity. Losing or maintaining weight were concerns for most of them. Young women used words like 'rolly', 'chubby', 'fat', and 'gross' to indicate the undesirable state that they mainly attributed to a lack of exercise or bad eating. This finding confirms how most participants adopted subject positions within the mainstream obesity discourse. The various narratives we heard about the 'healthy body' were stories constituted with elements of a dominant racist, sexist, heterosexist and ableist discourse of beauty. For instance Amar, one of the young South-Asian Canadian women, spoke of maintaining her weight and having a clear skin since 'that's what people see and I want it to be a healthy-looking face'. When asked what other practices she engaged in to feel 'healthy', she responded in the following manner:

Oh, tons of hair removal. Man, you name it, I've tried it. Waxing, tweezing. Right now, I'm getting electrolysis done, yup, on my eyebrows as well as upper lip area. I also bleach.

Here, Amar admitted to a number of practices including bleaching, a technique to lighten facial hair and skin that is quite well known among Canadian women of colour. Amar was not that different from other young women in that dominant (read colonial) constructions of white, heterosexual female attractiveness seemed to have real life consequences on their ideas of health and on their bodies. Attractiveness is invariably racialized and, in this study, the experiences of young women from the Asian-Canadian and Somali-Canadian communities were impacted by racist aesthetics. In an environment that associates beauty with being skinny, blonde and blue-eyed, they discursively constructed certain 'health' practices (health being defined their way) as important resources for social and occupational success.

DISCUSSION

This brief exploration of the narratives of young people in our study provides an understanding of how they constructed health using elements of dominant discourses of obesity, health, gender, sexuality, dis/ability and race. Overall, these young people constructed health in corporeal terms. They stressed being active, eating well and not being fat. This suggests a re-articulation of obesity discourse much like that found in studies of young people's meanings of health in New Zealand (Burrows, Wright and Jungersen-Smith 2003) and Australia (Wright, O'Flynn and Macdonald 2006). The prevalence of corporeal themes in the discursive construction of health is not surprising given their centrality within medical and mainstream messages about health in Canada. What is somewhat perplexing is the fact that participants in our study were well versed in the school and public health messages about nutrition and physical activity, but that their reported behaviours did not necessarily reflect that knowledge. Also, they generally constructed themselves as 'healthy' individuals, yet many acknowledged not doing the things they associated with health (e.g. regular physical activity, good nutrition). It seemed that, for the participants, health meant things that they considered inaccessible (fitness is too hard, sports are too expensive), irrelevant (they see themselves as fairly healthy), boring (walking, deliberate exercise, eating vegetables) or contradicting their tastes (no junk food, no TV, no video games). We could say that governmental and school imperatives aim to discipline and 'mark' the youthful body, to 'territorialize' it to use Deleuze and Guattari's (1983) concept. But this body is simultaneously fed by tastes and desires (often created by the mass media, commodity culture, peers) that continuously try to escape prescription. We could say that there is some resistance, as if this youthful body tended to de-territorialize its surface. In line with the territorializing attempts of the health education institutions, young people *speak* health as they see it (e.g. be physically active, eat well), but in opposition to the same attempts, they seldom *do* health.

But the notion of resistance can only be carried so far since participants were quite concerned about their bodily weight and shape, a discursive fragment that can easily be traced back to the dominant obesity discourse saturating their environment. In that sense, the participants were no different from other young Canadians. A larger survey by Health Canada (1999) found that achieving an ideal body weight and shape is one of the most important health issues among youth. Here, we must worry about the recitation of a discourse that emphasizes the importance of 'not being fat' and having a 'normal' body as such a discourse is particularly oppressive to corpulent or physically disabled youth whose bodies are often constructed in opposition to 'normality' and 'health'.

Not unrelated to this is the result concerning individual responsibility for one's health. Indeed, participants very much constructed health as something one does. This shows the extent to which participants recycled a healthist discourse that conceptualizes health as an individual and moral responsibility (Crawford 1980; Howell and Ingham 2001). The concern, here, is that the focus on the individual overshadows socio-cultural and environmental factors that affect health. In addition, such emphasis leads to the construction of illness and obesity as a failure in character, with the end-result of blaming those who fall short of maintaining health or weight

(Brandt and Rozin 1997; Colquhoun 1987). This may explain why, in the present study, youth with a mobility impairment resisted stereotypes of disability through 'performative acts' of the healthy body (e.g. they reported walking as much as they could, participating in adapted mainstream sports). Perhaps the most significant consequence of equating health with 'having a normal body' or 'not being fat' is the fact that our society has very restrictive and narrow ideas of 'normality'. While some participants mocked the importance of physical appearance and expressed their frustration with the masculine and feminine ideals, most confided that they strove for an 'ideal appearance', nonetheless. The problem is that this mode of being ultimately leads to uneasiness, shame or guilt since all young people may strive but very few will achieve the 'ideal' body.

Connecting health with outward appearance and notions of beauty is interesting in that some participants saw this as a pragmatic strategy with which to combat racialization, discrimination and marginalization. But it is, at the same time, problematic because constructing health in this manner may lead to some practices (e.g. young men taking supplements or drugs and young women splurging, fasting, dieting, tanning, waxing or bleaching) that do not seem particularly beneficial for the body. Indeed, youth are not exempt from being consumers of the commercialized products of a healthist culture. Since this culture provides discursive resources for making sense of health, youth constructed their own meanings of health and at the same time their own identities using these resources. They did so sometimes in subversive ways, but most often in a conformist fashion.

The participants' constructions of health were very much tied up with the larger discourses of conventional masculinity, femininity, and heteronormativity. Not all young people appropriated dominant ideology; on the contrary, quite a few showed important moments of resistance, for instance, by critiquing the media's conventional representations of gender or by mocking the social importance given to ideal male and female bodily forms. However, meanings of health as well as health practices seemed important to them as resources in their struggle to understand mainstream (i.e. 'Canadian', able-bodied, heterosexual) masculinity and femininity. For instance, young people of colour perceived the pervasive stereotypes and expectations regarding their gendered 'Asianness', 'South Asianness' or 'Somalianness' something that both males and females resisted. Males rearticulated dominant (i.e. what they see as 'Canadian') discourses of masculinity while some females spoke of their involvement in mainstream physical activity and 'health' practices. These are well known strategies (Cockerham, Rutten and Abel 1997; White, Young and Gillett 1995) to differentiate themselves from the 'Other' and to affirm their 'Canadianness'.

That being said, it is crucial to note that youth actively negotiated and resisted the different 'ways to be': they did not passively accept their 'identifications' (Weedon 1997) as 'woman' or 'disabled' or 'Somali-Canadian', but rather drew on discursive resources through which they could feel and understand their reality. Although we can see participants as constructed within discursive practices, they nonetheless exist as feeling and thinking subjects capable of resistance and innovation produced out of the confrontation of contradictory subject positions. Consider, for example, a young Somali-Canadian participant who had to negotiate a position within a discourse dominant in her Black, Muslim, Somali-Canadian community as well as a position within a discourse dominant among her mostly white, Christian, Euro-Canadian schoolmates. In general, participants could be seen as moving in and out of their various subject positions with considerable ease. In discussing health, they were generally involved in discursive practices that produced gender, race, or dis/ability as a reiteration of hegemonic norms, yet their performative acts also transpired fluidity and the possibility of interpellation by alternative discourses.

CONCLUSION

The poststructuralist approach used in this chapter has allowed for a conceptualization of young people as subjects who are interpellated by subject positions. Such positions exist at times within alternative discourses but mostly within the dominant obesity discourse, as it intersects with mainstream discourses of health, gender, sexuality, race and ability. This speaks to the power of discourses to structure subjectivity and experience. Indeed, it is at the crossroads of such discourses that young people constructed their (however temporary and fluid) subjectivity and position as 'healthy' subjects. Despite interesting moments of resistance, it is through the re-articulation of hegemonic understandings of the body and health that they constructed their simultaneous racial, ethnic, dis/ability, and gender identities.

Overall, these results speak to the importance of contesting current health promotion programs and writings, and of including alternative discourses that resist the construction of health in opposition to obesity, disability or marginalized status. Unless subversive discourses about health and obesity are given a more prominent place, young people's acquisition of new subject positions will remain limited, and health will remain elusive particularly for marginalized youth. For progressive change, we need to raise awareness about obesity discourse, its problematic discursive effects, and particularly how and why it constructs particular subjects.

Finally, it should be noted that health and physical education programs are producing messages that are well understood but often resisted by young people. The latter can *speak* health, as they construct it, but they seldom *do* health. Institutions are compelling the youthful body to obey, they are 'territorializing' it, but this body seems to retaliate. We are only now starting to map this process of territorialization and de-territorialization but the present findings point to the importance of shedding light on such processes and their intersection with gender, sexuality, race, culture and dis/ability. There is no doubt that research efforts in this direction are important but constitute only a small fraction of the work ahead of critical obesity scholars. Given discourses in popular culture surrounding obesity as well as the institutional and research practices that hold them in place, much is needed in terms of subversive scholarship to unsettle and challenge current notions of obesity, health and truth.

REFERENCES

Annis, N.M., Cash, T.F., and Hrabosky, J.I. (2004) 'Body image and psychosocial differences among stable average weight, currently overweight, and formerly overweight women: the role of stigmatizing experiences', *Body Image*, 1: 155–67.
Bartky, S.L. (1990) *Femininity and Domination: Studies in the Phenomenology of Oppression*, London: Routledge.
Bhabha, H.K. (1994) *The Location of Culture*, London: Routledge.
Boehmer, T., Lovegreen, S.L., Haire-Joshu, D. and Brownson, R.C. (2006) 'What constitutes an obesogenic environment in rural communities?', *American Journal of Health Promotion*, 20(6): 411–21.
Bordo, S. (1993) *Unbearable Weight: Feminism, Western Culture and the Body*, Berkeley: University of California Press.
Brandt, A.M. and Rozin, P. (eds) (1997) *Morality and Health*, New York: Routledge.
Braziel, J.E. and Lebesco, K. (eds) (2001) *Bodies Out of Bounds: Fatness and Transgression*, Berkeley: University of California Press.
Burrows, L. and Wright, J. (2004) 'The discursive production of childhood, identity and health', in J. Evans, B. Davies and J. Wright (eds) *Body Knowledge and Control: Studies in the Sociology of Education and Physical culture*, London: Routledge.
Burrows, L., Wright, J. and Jungersen-Smith, J. (2001) '"Look in the mirror and see how strong your muscles are . . .": New Zealand children's constructions of health and fitness', *Proceedings of the American Educational Research Association Annual Meeting*, Seattle, 10–14 April.
Butler, J. (1990) *Gender Trouble*, New York: Routledge.
———. (1997) *Excitable Speech: A Politics of the Performative*, New York: Routledge.
Campos, P. (2004) *The Obesity Myth: Why America's Obsession With Weight is Hazardous to Your Health*, New York: Penguin Books.
Campos, P., Saguy, A., Ernsberger, P., Oliver, E. and Gaesser, G. (2006) 'The epidemiology of overweight and obesity: public health crisis or moral panic?', *International Journal of Epidemiology*, 35(1): 55–60.
Cockerham, W.C., Rutten, A. and Abel, T. (1997) 'Conceptualizing contemporary health lifestyles: moving beyond Weber', *The Sociological Quarterly*, 38(2): 321–42.
Colquhoun, D. (1987) 'Health based physical education, the ideology of healthism and victim blaming', *British Journal of Physical Education*, 18: 5–13.
Crawford, R. (1980) 'Healthism and the medicalization of everyday life', *International Journal of Health Services*, 10(3): 365–88.
Deleuze, G. and Guattari, F. (1983) *Anti-oedipus: Capitalism and Schizophrenia*, Minneapolis: University of Minnesota Press.
Evans, J., Davies, B. and Wright, J. (2004) *Body Knowledge and Control: Studies in the Sociology of Physical Education and Health*, London: Routledge.

Evans, J., Rich, E., Allwood, R. and Davies, B. (2005) 'Fat fabrications', The British Journal of Teaching Physical Education, Winter.

Evans, J., Rich, E., and Davies, B. (2004) 'The emperor's new clothes: fat, thin and overweight. The social fabrication of risk and health', *Journal of Teaching Physical Education*, 23(4): 372–92.

Farrell, S.W., Braun, L., Barlow, C.E., Cheng, Y.J. and Blair, S.N. (2002) 'The relation of body mass index, cardiorespiratory fitness, and all-cause mortality in women', *Obesity Research*, 10: 417–23.

Flegal, K.M., Graubard, B.I., Williamson, D.F., and Gail, M.H. (2005) 'Excess deaths associated with underweight, overweight, and obesity', *Journal of the American Medical Association*, 293(15): 1861–7.

Foucault, M. (1973) *The Birth of the Clinic*, London: Tavistock.

———. (1978) *The History of Sexuality, Volume I: An Introduction*, Harmondsworth, England: Peregrine, Penguin Books.

———. (1979) *Discipline and Punish: The Birth of the Prison*, New York: Vintage.

Friedman, K.E., Reichmann, S.K., Costanzo, P.R., Zelli, A., Ashmore, J.A., and Musante, G.J. (2005) 'Weight stigmatization and ideological beliefs: relation to psychological functioning in obese adults', *Obesity Research* 13: 907–16.

Gaesser, G.A. (2003) 'Pro and con: is obesity a disease? (No)', *Family Practice News*, 33(16).

Gaesser, G.A. and Blair, S.N. (2002) *Big Fat Lies: The Truth About Your Weight and Your Health*, Carlsbad, CA: Gurze Books.

Gallagher, K. and Fusco, C. (2006) 'I.D.ology and the technologies of public (school) space: an ethnographic inquiry into the neo-liberal tactics of social (re)production', *Journal of Ethnography and Education*, 1(3): 301–18.

Gard, M. (2004) 'An elephant in the room and a bridge too far, or physical education and the "obesity epidemic"', in J. Evans, B. Davies and J. Wright (eds) *Body Knowledge and Control: Studies in the Sociology of Physical Education and Health*, London: Routledge.

Gard, M. and Wright, J. (2005) *The Obesity Epidemic: Science, Morality and Ideology*, London: Routledge.

Garland-Thomson, R. (2005) 'Feminist disability studies', *Signs: Journal of Women in Culture and Society*, 30: 1557–87.

George, T. and Rail, G. (2006) 'Barbie meets the Bindi: constructions of health among second generation South Asian Canadian women' *Journal of Women's Health and Urban Life*, 4(2): 45–67.

Grogan, S. (1999) *Body Image: Understanding Body Disaffection in Men, Women and Children*, London: Routledge.

Groskopf, B. (2005) 'The failure of bio–power: interrogating the "obesity crisis"', *Journal for the Arts, Sciences and Technology*, 3(1): 41–7.

Grosz, E. (1994) *Volatile Bodies: Towards a Corporeal Feminism*, Crows Nest, Australia: Allen and Unwin.

Halse, C. (2007) 'Bio-citizenship', paper presented at the international conference *Bio-Pedagogies: Schooling, Youth and the Body in the Obesity Epidemic*, Wollongong, Australia.

Health Canada (1999a) *Statistical Report on the Health of Canadians*, Ottawa: Available at: http://www.hc-sc.gc.ca/hppb/phdd/report/stat/eng/report.html.

Herrick, C. (2007) 'Risky bodies: public health, social marketing and the governance of obesity', *Geoforum*, 38(1): 90–102.

Holm, S. (2007) 'Obesity interventions and ethics', *Obesity Reviews*, 8(S1): 207–10.

Howell, J. and Ingham, A. (2001) 'From social problem to personal issue: the language of lifestyle', *Cultural Studies*, 15(2): 326–51.

Ikeda, J., Amy, N.K., Ernsberger, P., Gaesser, G.A., Berg, F.M., Clark, C.A., Parham, E.S. and Peters, P. (2005) 'The National Weight Control Registry: A critique', *Journal of Nutrition, Education and Behavior,* 37(4): 203–5.

Komesaroff, S. and Thomas, P.A. (2007) 'Combating the obesity epidemic: cultural problems demand cultural solutions', *Internal Medicine Journal,* 37(5): 287.

Lang, T. and Rayner, G. (2007) 'Overcoming policy cacophony on obesity: an ecological public health framework for policymakers', *Obesity Reviews,* 8(S1): 165–81.

Lupton, D. (1992) 'Discourse analysis: a new methodology for understanding the ideologies of health and illness', *Australian Journal of Public Health,* 16: 145–50.

MacNeill, M. and Rail, G. (2007) 'Youth obesity, health literacy and biopedagogy', presentation made at the annual *North American Society for the Sociology of Sport* conference, Pittsburgh, USA, November.

Mark, D. (2005) 'Deaths attributable to obesity', *Journal of the American Medical Association,* 293(15): 1918–19.

Miah, A. and Rich, E. (2006) *The Medicalisation of Cyberspace,* London: Routledge.

Minh–Ha, T.T. (1995) 'Writing postcoloniality and feminism', in B. Ashcroft, G. Griffiths and H. Tifflin (eds) *The Postcolonial Studies Reader,* New York: Routledge.

Monaghan, L.F. (2007) 'McDonaldizing men's bodies? Slimming, associated (ir)rationalities and resistances', *Body and Society,* 13(2): 67–93.

———. (2008) 'Men, physical activity, and the obesity discourse: critical understandings from a qualitative study', *Sociology of Sport Journal,* 25(1): 97–129.

Murray, S. (2007) 'Corporeal knowledges and deviant bodies: perceiving the fat body', *Social Semiotics,* 17(3): 361–73.

———. (2008) 'Pathologizing "fatness": medical authority and popular culture', *Sociology of Sport Journal,* 25(1): 7–21.

Nestle, M. (2002) *Food Politics: How the Food Industry Influences Nutrition and Health,* Berkeley: University of California Press.

Oliver, J.E. (2005) *Fat Politics: The Real Story Behind America's Obesity Epidemic,* Oxford: Oxford University Press.

———. (2006) 'The politics of pathology: how obesity became an epidemic disease', *Perspectives in Biology and Medicine,* 49(4): 611–27.

Orbach, S. (1988) *Fat is a Feminist Issue,* London: Arrow Books.

Rail, G. (2002) 'Postmodernism and sport studies', in J. Maguire and K. Young (eds) *Perspectives in the Sociology of Sport,* London, England: Elsevier Press.

Rail, G., Beausoleil, N., MacNeill, M., Burrows, L. and Wright, J. (2003) *Canadian Youth's Discursive Constructions of Fitness and Health,* Grant proposal to (and research funded by) the Social Sciences and Humanities Research Council of Canada.

Rail, G. and Harvey, J. (1995) 'Body at work: Michel Foucault and the sociology of sport', *Sociology of Sport Journal,* 12(2): 165–80.

Raphael, D. (2003) 'Addressing the social determinants of health in Canada: bridging the gap between research findings and public policy', *Policy Options,* March: 35–44.

Rich, E. and Evans, J. (2005) 'Fat ethics: the obesity discourse and body politics', *Social Theory and Health,* 3(4): 341–58.

Saguy, A. and Almeling, R. (2008) 'Fat in the fire? Science, the news media, and the "obesity epidemic"', *Sociological Forum,* 22(1): 53–83.

Spivak, G.C. (1995) 'Can the subaltern speak?', in B. Ashcroft, G. Griffiths and H. Tiffin (eds) *The Post-colonial Studies Reader,* London and New York: Routledge.

Vertinsky, P. (2004) '"Power geometries": disciplining the gendered body in the spaces of the War Memorial Gym', in P. Vertinsky and S. McKay (eds) *Disciplining Bodies in the Gymnasium: Memory, Monument, Modernism*, London: Routledge.

Weedon, C. (1997) *Feminist Practice and Poststructuralist Theory*, London: Blackwell.

White, P., Young, K. and Gillett, J. (1995) 'Bodywork as a moral imperative: some critical notes on health and fitness', *Society and Leisure*, 18(1): 159–82.

Wilkinson, R. and Marmot, M. (1998) *Social Determinants of Health: The Solid Facts*, Copenhagen: World Health Organization.

World Health Organization (WHO) (2000) *Obesity: Preventing and Managing the Global Epidemic. WHO Technical Report Series 894*, Geneva: World Health Organization.

———. (2006) *Obesity*. Online. Available HTTP: http://www.who.int/topics/obesity/en/ (accessed 24 July 2008).

Wright, J. (1995) 'A feminist poststructuralist methodology for the study of gender construction in physical education: description of a study', *Journal of Teaching in Physical Education*, 15(1): 1–24.

———. (2001) 'Gender reform in physical education: a poststructuralist perspective', *Journal of Physical Education New Zealand*, 34(1): 15–25.

Wright, J., O'Flynn, G. and Macdonald, D. (2006) 'Being fit and looking healthy: young women's and men's constructions of health and fitness', *Sex Roles*, 54: 707–716.

Wright, J., Rail, G., MacDonald, D., MacNeill, M. and Evans, J. (2006) *Bio-Pedagogies: Schooling, Youth, the Body and the "Obesity Epidemic"*, unpublished grant proposal to the International Studies and Alliances Committee, University of Wollongong, Australia.

11 Performative Health in Schools
Welfare Policy, Neoliberalism and Social Regulation?

Emma Rich and John Evans

INTRODUCTION

> . . . social control, social surveillance and social welfare are becoming increasingly harder to distinguish.
>
> (Fitzpatrick 2001: 192)

Fitzpatrick's observations concerning the blurring of the boundaries between welfare and control are the focus of this chapter, as we examine such a process in relation to anti childhood obesity policy in schools in the UK. In schools across western societies, curricular and pedagogies are being drastically re-shaped by initiatives and policies concerned with tackling a childhood 'obesity epidemic' (Evans, Rich, Davies and Allwood 2008; Burrows 2007). In England and Wales, central Government has sought joint action from its agencies, the Department of Health (DoH) and the Department for Education and Skills (DfES; renamed the Department for Children, Schools and Families in 2007), to address health matters through policy affecting the whole environment of schools. Many of these initiatives are being implemented as part of a Public Services Agreement Target: to halt, by 2010, 'the year-on-year increase in obesity among children under 11' in the context of a broader strategy to tackle obesity in the population as a whole (DoH 2004). In an effort to monitor and regulate childhood obesity, young people are now being subjected to an increasing range of techniques of surveillance, which involve not only monitoring their lifestyles in and outside schools (e.g., their food choices, physical activity levels) but more directly the collection of information on their individual bodies with a view to monitoring and altering their weight and size.

In this chapter, we argue that the proliferation of these techniques and policies are part of a wider biopolitical culture of social governance via the direct surveillance of young people's lives within the UK. Following Penna (2005: 143), we suggest that these interventions form part of a political project which involves 'the use of surveillance as a mode of societal governance' supported and intensified by developments in technologies which monitor bodies (for example the development of pedometers, biometric technology for fingerprint screening or advances in digital culture (see Miah and Rich 2008). Such techniques have developed at a time when:

> the issue of surveillance is given renewed importance through the discourses surrounding the proliferation of 'control' technologies and the rhetoric of (in)security pervading contemporary politics.
>
> (Ajana 2005)

We outline how anti-obesity policy forms part of this wider political project towards the social governance of young people and the management of societal change above and beyond the need to protect the population from ill health. As outlined in previous chapters, obesity has typically been constructed as a 'crisis' of potentially catastrophic proportions. Burrows and Wright (2007), for example, refer to the way in which such unbounded crises make it easier to talk about intervening in the lives of ever younger children and in ever more drastic ways. This representation of obesity as 'crisis' has resulted in a range of policies directed at the social and material environments of schools all of which are constructed within a discursive frame that invokes a curious (and contradictory) mix of welfare and neoliberal ideals. While the former celebrate care, protection and social responsibility through regulation and intervention, the latter laud individualism, autonomy, freedom from constraint and independent action on the part of the individual. Reflecting such ideals, anti-obesity policy has in recent years been radically interventionist. On the one hand, presaging adaptations both to the school environment (for example, changing school lunch menus, advocating the removal of vending machines and changes to curricular, etc.) and to 'the body' via intrusive forms of information retrieval involving the measurement and assessment of body size, weight and shape. On the other hand, however, such measures have been couched in a language affirming that 'ultimately' individuals (and their families) are blameworthy, should be more disciplined and take greater responsibility for their parlous state of health. Herein lies the 'biopolitics' of childhood obesity reflecting the coexistence of two modalities of power: control and discipline (see Ajana 2005).

In the final part of the chapter, we examine how these technologies of governance 'translate into principles of communication' and become *pedagogised* within school contexts leaving little obvious space for resistance amongst the young people who are subjected to them. We suggest that school based 'health interventions' can have damaging and enduring effects on the health and well being of some young people, especially the vulnerable and those whose cultural values are at variance with those of the school. We explore how, given the total pedagogisation of obesity discourse across whole school environments, and the hierarchical manner in which pedagogical activity occurs, there is very little space or opportunity for young people to resist the pervasive influence of biopedagogies. Moreover, we examine the severity to which young people may experience biopedagogies as a central and damaging feature of their school lives. To do so, we draw upon data collected from over forty young women diagnosed with anorexia nervosa or other eating disorders who were resident at a leading centre in the UK for the treatment of eating disorders. Although the centre catered for both males and females no boys were available for interview, and thus only young women were involved in the study. The interviews formed part of a wider ethnographic project exploring the relationship between education and the aetiology of eating disorders (see Evans et al. 2008). The young women whose voices are heard in this paper are aged between eleven and eighteen, come from 'middle class families', and all have attended what might be described as 'high status' comprehensive, grammar, or private, secondary schools. All the study participants had been diagnosed with anorexia or bulimia, and were judged by the clinic to be at different stages of 'illness' or recovery, but each was suffering in sufficient severity to warrant residential treatment and care.

CHILDHOOD OBESITY POLICY: TOWARDS SOCIAL GOVERNANCE?

It is important to note that 'attempts to exercise governance take place through a particular discursive construction of children and their protection' (Penna 2005: 143). Health education policies in the UK are invariably underpinned by a broader narrative of risk espousing the need for protection (against death, disease, ill health, etc) and are legitimated via moral panics concerning the prevalence and extent of childhood obesity, nurtured by media (TV, newspaper and film) reporting and bioscience research (see Gard and Wright 2005). The construction of obesity as a serious threat to populations in certain respects exemplifies Foucault's (1976) notion of bio-power which on the surface works in the interest of humankind to prevent the demise of 'man-as-species' but simultaneously serves other social functions, namely, to control and regulate 'deviant' populations. The construction of obesity as a crisis that threatens the future lives of our childhood population reflects the 'governmental preoccupation with social welfare and security, the large scale management of life and death in the interests of the state' (Howell 2007: 293). Obesity is constructed as a crisis of global proportions with potentially fatal consequences, from which populations, particularly the young, need state protection. In this view, as populations have grown and become more fluid and complex, nation states have become 'more concerned about the management of life (bio-power) and the governing of populations' (Howson 2004: 125), particularly in relation to health, disease, sexuality, welfare and education. Thus populations become objects of 'surveillance, analysis, intervention and correction across space and time' (Nettleton 1992, quoted in Howson 2004: 125).

With the construction of obesity as a global crisis, the political context is set for state intervention and welfare policy to 'protect' young people from the growing epidemic. Indeed, the role of what has been coined 'the nanny state' and welfare, commonly resurfaces in discussions around childhood obesity policy in both the UK and beyond. In America for example, Brownell and Horgen (2004: 123) suggest enacting 'a small state or national tax on soft drinks, snack foods and fast foods, earmarking the money for schools'. However such 'fat tax' measures have been severely attacked by neoliberal and traditional conservatives who saw it as anti free markets and an example of 'nanny state' politics (see Gard in this book). In the UK it is even mooted that children should be removed from parents if they fail to effectively regulate and monitor their offspring's eating behaviour and weight. For example, on February 27th 2007 the *Daily Mirror*, a popular British tabloid, reported the case of an 'overweight 8 year old, weighing 218 pounds', purportedly 'four times the weight of a "healthy" child of his age'. His mother feared she might lose custody unless he lost weight and was allowed to keep him only after striking a deal with social workers to safeguard his welfare. The child was in danger of being placed on the childcare register simply, it seemed, for being 'too fat'. Such cases reflect the fearsome, medical research-informed authority that 'obesity discourse' and those who espouse it now possess to define how populations should 'read' illness and health, and be rehabilitated should they not accept its messages (Evans et al. 2008). In this way, obesity discourse connects with a wider orientation within welfare policies which constructs children (or to be more exact, those of certain social class and culture) as always potentially 'at risk' and in need of protection, and legitimates the need for state intervention for the child's welfare, be this through placing the child in care, the need for national action via taxation, or the proliferation of policies oriented towards creating healthy schools and surveying young people's bodies. As will be revealed below, increasingly, information about young people's bodies, weight, diets and lifestyles are being collected through school-based interventions. This discourse of protection from future ill health within such policy is significant because simultaneously it serves other functions; it is 'never simply about technical issues of this or that situation and constituency' (Penna 2005: 144) but, in the case of health and obesity, is always grounded in broader discourses concerning citizenship, fat phobia, and racialization (see Chapter 13, this volume). This process of racialization, is not 'an ideological use of racism, but a state racism which is implicit in biopolitical societies' (Kelly 2004: 61).

Whilst on the surface, these policies appear to be oriented towards protecting young people from ill health, their ulterior goal is not only to rescue a child population 'at risk' but to regulate 'deviant' populations by announcing and (re)establishing acceptable social norms. Indeed, anti-obesity policies are part of wider political strategies 'which do not have as their central focus either meeting the needs of children or responding to child abuse, but the assessment and management of risk' (Parton 1998). As Penna (2005: 144) notes:

[W]elfare programmes are intrinsically embedded in political projects, projects that are concerned with managing societal change and that are rooted in normative perceptions of what constitutes desirable social development. Welfare policies, in this sense, are technologies of governance: they are vehicles through which visions of the 'good society' are steered.

In the emotionally loaded language of obesity discourse, the term 'epidemic,' and the specific construction of obesity as an 'unbounded crisis' (Gard and Wright 2005) function discursively to both rationalise and legitimate the various forms of surveillance of, and information gathering upon, young people's bodies. This language not only curtails critique of such interventions (for who in their right mind would contest measures to check the rampant spread of 'disease') but also paralyses more searching analyses of the antecedents of ill health. These linguistic tendencies and techniques are evident in the obesity report released in October 2007 in the UK by the Foresight Commission (Foresight 2007). Sanctioned by central Government this Report is particularly important because it will not only define thinking and practice on obesity/health issues for some years to come in the UK and elsewhere but also, once recycled globally through obesity networks, sanction unprecedented levels of monitoring and surveillance from cradle to grave, in and outside schools. As we have elsewhere pointed out (Evans et al. 2008), Foresight (2007) offers an example *par excellence* of contemporary health discourse; its terms amounting to 'a paradigm shift' on earlier explanations of the 'obesity crisis' and a step towards change in thinking on 'intervention'. The Foresight Report, *Tackling Obesities—Future projects*, made headline grabbing news with the claim that obesity was 'as bad as climate risk' and that 50 percent of the population would become obese in the next 24 years. Typically, the Report articulated its message through a language and vocabulary of risk and mortality, in this instance suggesting that obesity risks are on the scale of 'global warming'. Clearly its narrative was intended not just to scare populations but rationalise and sanction new strategies involving unprecedented levels of intervention, surveillance, monitoring and control, reaching into every aspect of our private and public lives:

> The pace of the technological revolution is outstripping human evolution and, for an increasing number of people, weight gain is the inevitable—and largely involuntary—consequence of exposure to a modern lifestyle. This is not to dismiss personal responsibility altogether, but to highlight a reality: that the forces that drive obesity are, for many people, overwhelming. Although what we identify in this report as 'passive obesity' occurs across all population groups, the socially and economically disadvantaged and some ethnic minorities are more vulnerable.
>
> (Foresight 2007: 5)

As we've pointed out elsewhere (Evans et al. 2008) in this carefully framed version of environmental and biological determinism, we are all deemed to reside in an 'obesiogenic environment' and, as 'we' are all subject to biological frailty, we are all potentially 'passively obese', fat by default. Thus are the conditions set for reinstating obesity as a matter of welfare and for cradle to grave intervention into the actions of communities, families, parents, pupils, teachers and the practices of food producers and advertisers, in effect reaching into every aspect of our private and pubic lives.

However, in this, and other policies oriented towards obesity, the paradox of integrating welfare notions of protecting the child from the risks of ill health (and the 'obesogenic' environment) while nurturing neoliberal individualism and the fabrication of the individually active/agentic 'globally available fit (slender/muscular) body' (see Chapter 13, this volume) become all too evident. This discursive formation simultaneously constructs a need for protection and intervention strategies, whilst also inciting individual action and the burden of responsibility on individuals. For example, the Foresight Report facilitates not only the celebration of a particularly narrow (white ableist, middle-class) set of corporeal virtues concerning slenderness and the relentless pursuit of 'being thin', a vision endorsed in subsequent Health Reports (Smith 2007) but also implicitly endorses the view that bad biology, psychology and habits, resulting in too little exercise and over indulgence in the pleasures of readily available, cheap, bad food, can be apportioned disproportionately to particular categories of the population, thereby, perpetuating a culture in which selected individuals (and their families) can be singled out, 'othered' and held ultimately responsible for not achieving these ideals (Evans et al. 2008). Indeed, despite the apparent welfarist orientations of 'state intervention' and 'social care', and the focus on 'obesogenic environments', ironically, the most invidious feature of obesity discourse, endemic in media reporting and implicit in this and other policy texts remains—is the idea that health problems are essentially the fault of certain individuals (especially the poor, working class and ethnic minorities).

PERFORMATIVE HEALTH AND THE PEDAGOGIZATION OF SURVEILLANCE IN SCHOOLS

The pedagogization of these forms of surveillance and the activation of disciplinary techniques in schools, is one expression of the biopolitics of childhood obesity in schools; it indicates 'that the two modalities of power (discipline and control) are not mutually exclusive but coexist within the working of biopolitics and through the hybridisation of management techniques' (Ajana 2005). We would add, they are also present in the hybridisation of technologies used to gather information on children's weight and shape—a point to which we will later return.

Drawing upon Ball's (2005) concept of performativity, we argue that Government policies on health education in schools have become increasingly performative in nature by focusing on factors such as comparison measurement, assessment and accountability. In Ball's (2003) terms, performativity is a technology, a culture and a mode of regulation that employs judgements, comparisons and displays as means of incentive, control, attrition and change—based on rewards and sanctions (both material and symbolic). The performances (of individual subjects or organizations) serve as measures of productivity or output, or displays of 'quality', or 'moments' of promotion or inspection. As such they stand for, encapsulate or represent the worth, quality or value of an individual or organization within a field of judgement.

Thus we find ourselves with the rather odd idea that health is relevant only in so far as it can be measured and evidenced in institutions like schools, which have a putative capacity to ensure that students (and their guardians) achieve specific goals, such as weight loss, proper diet and exercise regimens. The combined effect of which is a standardized approach to health that is both medicalized and narrowly focused on that which can be easily measured and assessed. This results in what we have termed 'performative health'.

Performative health policies are imbued with technologies of governance that steer particular school populations towards medicalized and objectified norms concerning weight management (usually in the direction of 'weight loss'). They do so, not simply by the direct regulation and surveillance of young people's bodies in schools, but also via more subtle, but less certain, forms of control involving a combination of mass surveillance and self regulation, which Foucault (1977, 1980) called 'disciplinary power'. In this process individuals and populations are ascribed responsibility for regulating and looking after themselves, though often according to criteria over which they have very little say or control while, at the same time, being more or less relentlessly monitored in their capacity to do so, in some respects from cradle to grave (see Foresight 2007; Evans et al. 2008). Performative health is, in this sense, not simply enforced in schools, but forms part of, and endorses, the pedagogization of obesity discourse exercised as *body pedagogies* (Evans and Davies 2005, Evans et al. 2008) or body pedagogics (Shilling 2005, 2008) and their specific variants in schools. In this sense, technologies of information gathering upon and of young people's bodies act not only to measure (and control) them, but more directly to regulate (and discipline) them. Techniques of data gathering on and through the body also impart a particular judgement about the individual, and his or her 'chosen' lifestyle. They not only function as data gathering techniques, but also implore young people to participate in the self-monitoring and self-disciplining of their own and others' bodies.

THE FAT TAG: THE INFORMATIONALIZATION OF YOUNG PEOPLE'S BODIES

The range of techniques available to gather information in schools related to the status of young people's health is ever increasing. These technologies include fingerprint screening to monitor young people's lunch choices, regular weighing to determine a BMI classification, the use of pedometers to count the number of steps a child will take, skinfold measurements, heart rate monitors, lunch box inspections and dietary constraints. The standardisation of the body through performative health thus is both rendered possible and consolidated by these various forms of quasi-medical assessment. Together they nurture 'a culture and mode of regulation' itself 'a system of measures, and indicators (signs) and sets of relationships' in which individuals (teachers and pupils) are compelled to fabricate 'versions of themselves' in order to meet ideal expectations, 'fit in' and 'do well'. Many of the young women we interviewed, reported that such techniques were critical moments in how they came to view their own bodies. They represented experiences which, propelled some towards drastic forms of dietary restraint:

> We used to have to get weighed in the class and that was terrible [. . .] It was to do with maths or something . . . and that was horrible . . . because then everybody knew your weight and then . . . a lot of the lads actually used to go on . . . and . . . you know . . . shouting out your weight in the class . . . things like that . . . that was terrible . . . really terrible. (Rebekah, interview)
>
> I used to be overweight and I remember one time at school when the whole class got weighed and the teacher said "oh it's the big one" and I was the heaviest in the year! (Lara, poster)

Although recent reports and policies advocate more sensitive approaches to weighing in schools, they nonetheless justify such actions by the need to follow the physical development of children, prevent possible medical problems, associated with obesity, detect any deviation from 'normal' development and correct aberrant behaviour. Research has reported other forms of surveillance that extend into the daily lives of young people. Lunch time inspections of food boxes and choices are now frequently undertaken by teachers (O'Neill 2004; and see Chapter 12, this volume) in schools. Elsewhere, in Australia, Leahy and Harrison (2003) have documented the phenomenon known as 'fat laps' in primary schools, where children identified as exceeding recommended body weight norms were required to run around the school field in their lunchtimes.

These techniques have to be situated within a 'society in which surveillance is rapidly becoming the technology of choice in configuring new modes of social governance' (Penna 2005: 149). In the UK, they fall within a wider policy framework focused on protecting young people from risk. For example, in 2003, the Government published a green paper called *Every Child Matters* (ECM) following the death of Victoria Climbié, a young girl who was horrifically abused and tortured, and eventually killed by her great aunt and the man with whom they lived in England. This horrific event led to extensive discussion about protection of young people and the role of children's services. ECM sets out five key outcomes for children and young people including: being healthy, staying safe, enjoying and achieving, making a positive contribution to society and achieving economic wellbeing. To achieve this, the focus has been on ensuring that organisations providing services to children, including health professionals and schools, take a more integrated approach to Care:

> The long term aim is to build on these developments to integrate information across services and ensure professionals share concerns at an early stage. To achieve this, we want to see a local information hub developed in every authority consisting of a list of all the children living in their area and basic details.
>
> (DfES 2003: 52–53)

However, ECM went much further than change and improvement to the child protection system: as initially conceived, it reached into every agency and avenue of child welfare, including education. The Victoria Climbié inquiry report by Lord Laming (2003) made clear that child protection could not be 'separated from polices to improve children's lives as a whole'. He wrote, 'We need to focus on the universal services as a whole—designed to protect children and to maximise their potential'. Consequently, the *Every Child Matters* policy sought to establish:

> a framework for services that cover children and young people from birth to 19 living in England [. . .] It aims to reduce the number of children who experience educational failure, engage in offending or anti-social behaviour, suffer ill health, or become teenage parents.
>
> (DfES 2003: 6)

By dissolving boundaries between service providers, for example, of health care and education, *ECM* not only extended the range of agencies in which pedagogical activity and surveillance routinely occurred, but simultaneously regulated the behaviours of all those involved in those settings through setting targets and outcomes for institutions and individuals to achieve. Indeed, many of the anti-obesity measures in the UK, are formed under the *Every Child Matters* policy, including the Government setting targets for food standards, and for healthy schools in relation to student health.

Throughout the development of these policies, new technologies have been utilised as a way to monitor and regulate risk factors to protect young people. The Children's Act 2004[1], quickly followed *ECM* in the UK, granting the UK Government power to set up an electronic database that tracks children in England and Wales known as Contact Point. This was established under The Children Act 2004 Information Database (England) Regulations 2007 which allows the details of every child in England and Wales to be held on an electronic database. In addition to basic information on a child's name, address, their parents or guardians, information will also be collected on each government service they use, including those associated with health (GP, NHS in full etc). Other tracking systems seek to identity 'vulnerable children before they get to the point of offending' (Penna 2005). For example, the Government Web Based Scheme RYOGENS (Reducing Youth Offending Generic National Solution (www.ryogens.org.uk) claims to be a web based system 'that helps practitioners from different agencies to share information about children in a safe and secure manner' in relation to crime prevention' (Government Forum 2008). The utilisation of technology to advance ways to monitor and regulate 'risk' has also been utilised in relation to the tracking and regulation of childhood obesity. In 2005, the National Child Measuring Programme was introduced, which legislates that every year, children in reception (4–5 years) and year 6 (10–11 years old) are weighed and measured in school. This information not only informs local services, but is used as surveillance data to monitor and analyse trends in growth patterns and obesity. In November 2007, the Government introduced the Health and Social Care Bill, which made legislative changes to the NCMP. Under the new provisions, all parents of children in Reception and Year 6 who take part in the NCMP will receive their child's results. In addition to this, parents will be given a letter giving them advice about their child's results and directed to an Internet Web site to regularly calculate their child's BMI.

The use of digital technology such as electronic databases, or the Internet, to aid social surveillance of young people is therefore becoming an ubiquitous feature of welfare policy in the UK. As Miah and Rich (2008) observe, changes in digital culture have brought about different mechanisms through which medicalisation and governance might take place. In their account of the ways in which the Internet and Web are impacting medical discourse, and health culture, they argue that the Internet has provided a range of technologies which facilitate the sort of regulation being advocated in the 'parental alert' letters about children's BMI. Online BMI calculators such as the ones being advocated in letters to parents, allow users to enter their height and weight details, which will then generate a BMI classification. Similarly, advances in biometric technology are now being utilised whereby schools can take the fingerprints of children to monitor lunch choices. Perhaps more controversially, as DNA testing and genetic technologies (see Rich and Miah 2006) continue to develop, the scope for screening and surveillance may become increasingly intrusive and offer new modes of governance. Advances in information technology such as these impact upon the nature of surveillance, although it does not signal the 'redundancy of previous modes of discipline and control' (Ajar 2005).

Weighing, alongside other initiatives, is not simply an exercise in informing young people about their health, but a mechanism for achieving an assessed outcome. Much like academic performance, under the guise of improving young people's health, we see a form of liberal governance which produces particular *affects* amongst young people, especially some young women: anxiety, stress and guilt. They effect a form of social engineering in which agencies can reach into the lives of young people, through pedagoziation both within the school, and now beyond into family relationships (for example, via the requirement for parents to monitor their child's weight online). Moreover, these techniques involve 'the use of surveillance as a mode of societal governance' (Penna 2005: 143) that becomes incredibly difficult for young people to resist, given that it is infused with moral judgements as to how they 'ought' to be. Through disciplinary mechanisms, young people's bodies are standardised as they are coded, weighed, monitored, regulated and classified. Within our research we have reported that such policies confer considerable power onto teachers and other health educators, not only in terms of the access to information they collect around young people's bodies, but also the way they can shape bodies. One of our participants, Anne, recalled that, despite beginning to feel weak from her extreme dieting, teachers continued to emphasise the need for her to 'push herself' in terms of physical activity:

> Emmm . . . they just sort of said 'push yourselves to the limit' . . . and I thought . . . you know . . . I sort of didn't kind of think I was fit enough sometimes . . . [. . .] . . . near the end . . . you know . . . I was quite weak . . . and they . . . and they sort of made you push yourselves to the limit and I was like 'help I can't do this!'
>
> (Anne, interview)

In addition to this teachers are given licence to bestow moral judgements upon young people's bodies, as Lydia, one of our respondents commented:

> She (teacher) picked out this girl who was literally like this thick (pointing to a pole in the room) and she said 'now this looks like a girl who is the right weight'. That really upset me because I just thought I have to get (my weight) down quick, so yeah that probably had a big effect on me.
>
> (Lydia, interview)

Many of these types of alarming commentaries made by teachers were legitimated by a narrative of welfare and protection of young people, of the need to intervene in order to protect the child's future well-being:

> I think it made me a bit worse . . . there was the teacher . . . she was saying like stuff like to all the pupils like 'oh you're all so lucky at the moment, you can eat like horses but you'll all be really fat when you're older if you carry on eating like this.
>
> (Jane, interview)

Here, then, we see the interpellation of the individual body, with the preferred/ideal 'species' implicit in obesity discourse. Biopolitics affords teachers the apparatus to pedagogise the need for young people to work 'autonomously' on their *individual* body, in order to address the broader risks pertinent to 'man-as-species'. These practices not only homogenise young people's health and bodies, but often leave them powerless to resist the normalising effects on their bodies and choices they make: 'If I see someone having something healthier than me I immediately feel guilty as I feel I am eating so much fat and it disgusts me' (Ruth, interview).

For these young women, escaping the normalising effects associated with representations of weight was incredibly difficult. As we have elsewhere illustrated (Evans et al 2008; Evans and Davies 2006; Rich and Evans 2005) the pressures to evaluate and judge their own and others' bodies against unattainable social ideals and of routinely being evaluated, judged and displayed were ever present across all features of schooling. Lunch-times, for example, were described as virulent environments in which the girls routinely surveyed not only their own, but also others' behaviour: 'Not many people were eating like a proper lunch so there was no way I was going to' (Viki, interview).

The message these young women hear is that they are to take control of their health by making 'healthy choices', particularly in relation to diet:

> You just learn that some things are good for you and some things are bad and should be avoided. That's why I find it so hard here when they put a pasty in front of you because I just think 'fat'. You don't learn that there are other things in 'bad' foods that are also good for you, like protein and carbohydrates. (Lauren, interview)

Our data illustrate how normalisation is incorporated into body peda-gogies to produce particular understandings and representations of one's body. The young women's narratives reveal that as they experience instruction around health and exercise, they are also learning to regulate their own bodies and weight and make judgements on others. As Burrows and Wright (2007) suggest, children and young people are being offered a number of ways to understand and change themselves, and take action to change others and their environments. By defining whose and what bodies have status and value, 'body pedagogies' also constitute acts of inclusion and exclusion. They also carry particularly strong moral overtones in the notions of the body they prescribe and define, an individual's character and value, their sense of self, can be judged essentially in terms of 'weight', size or shape. The 'overweight' body then represents an individual's moral failure to fulfil the requirements of neo-liberal subjectivity since fatness comes to represent a self that is lazy, self-indulgent and lacking control. This representation produces hierarchies of the body relating to size, shape and weight, and renders the disciplinary techniques of obesity discourse as self generated and self produced. In the case of obesity, biopower and disciplinary techniques are particularly effective because forms of surveillance are often interpreted by those subjected to them, through 'common sense' frameworks and ideologies about exercise, weight and health.

CONCLUSION: OBSCURING THE INTERSECTIONALITY OF WEIGHT AND HEALTH

In this chapter we have argued that there has been a rapid growth in instruments of surveillance that collect data on and through young people's bodies. Concomitantly, this has invoked particular forms of disciplinary practice that are difficult for young people (perhaps especially the white middle class) to resist. This is not to suggest that young people are cultural dupes, indeed they always and invariably recontexualize health knowledge through their own 'knower structures' (Maton 2006). Moreover, in work elsewhere (Rich and Evans 2007) we have explored how the young women with anorexia we interviewed were both complicit and resistant to performative health. However, for many of these women, the spaces for resistance are ultimately and ironically through their hybrid anorexic bodies.

The pervasiveness of these health imperatives not only impact on pupils. Teachers and other school staff find they now have to meet the expectations of inspection and appraisal regimes and work on persons and populations to achieve 'their transformational and disciplinary impact' (Shore and Wright 1999, quoted in Ball 2004: 152). In other words, seemingly apolitical health policies such as these are political projects in themselves, grounded in broader ideals about changes and developments in societies and the types of bodies and performances that are to be valued. Certain populations are privileged in the process while others are marginalised and considered culpable or deviant (the wrong shape, size and weight) by default. At its worst, reductionist and essentialist orientations of the body within this discourse, lead to a biopolitical homogenising of the class, gendered and raced complexities of conditions such as obesity. This reflects a 'biopolitical state racism' (Foucault 2003) imbued in state concerns with the control of biological processes.

The emergence of policies concerned with addressing childhood obesity can, then, be understood not simply as a technical motion to address ill-health, but a project bound up in wider climate of welfare policies that govern and regulate modern societies (Clarke 2004; Fitzpatrick 2001; Penna 2005). In the UK, where tracking and monitoring are now a feature of wider welfare policies, particularly since the Children Act 2004, obesity policies continue to gain momentum as a form of governance. These policies facilitate action, and self-regulation of those it targets, and in doing so, tends to depoliticise the complex intersections that concern health and weight.

The discursive presentation of these policies and initiatives not only obscures and depoliticises young people's social rights but obstructs discussion about the socio-economic and-cultural complexities that are a central feature of obesity. The co-option of wider health concerns into pedagogical practice, places young people under constant surveillance, and presses them towards monitoring their bodies; not through coercion but by facilitating *knowledge* around 'obesity' related risks/issues and 'instructing' them on how to eat healthily, stay active and lose weight. The racialized, classed and gendered specificities of these discourses are tied to the ways in which the promotion of the ideal feminine body as disciplined, normalised and slender, has been historically rooted to a middle class femininity that is specifically tied to whiteness (see Azzarito in this book; Oliver and Lalik 2004; Seid 1989). Indeed the production of these discourses through neo-liberal ideals where the individual is responsible for adopting a healthy life-style, glosses over the many health disparities that exist not only between socio economic groups, but between different ethnicities.

NOTES

1. See Penna (2005) for an analysis of the passage of the Children Act through Parliament, and of section 12 that facilitates the establishment electronic databases to track the progress of all children in England and Wales.

REFERENCES

Ajana, B. (2005) 'Surveillance and biopolitics', *Electronic Journal of Sociology*, 7, retrieved 22 July 2008, from http://www.sociology.org/content/2005/tier1/ajana_biopolitics.pdf

Ball, S. J. (2003) 'The teacher's soul and the terrors of performativity', *Journal of Education Policy*, 18(2): 215–228

Ball, S. J. (2004) *Professionalism, Managerialism and Performativity*, London: Institute of Education, University of London.

Brownell, K. D., and Horgen. K. B. (2004) *Food Fight: The Inside Story of the Food Industry, America's Obesity Crisis, and What We Can Do About It*, Chicago: Contemporary Books.

Burrows, L. (2007) 'Kiwi Kids are Weetbix kids: Body matters in health education', a paper presented at Performative Health and Body Pedagogies: every child matters, Society for Education Studies and Loughborough University one day seminar. Loughborough.

Burrows, L. and Wright, J. (2007) 'Prescribing practices: Shaping healthy children in schools', *International Journal of Children's Rights*, 15: 83–98.

Clarke, J. (2004) *Changing Welfare, Changing States*, Sage: London.

Department of Health (2004) *Choosing Health: Making Healthy Choices Easier*, White Paper, London: DoH Publications Orderline.

DfES (2003) *Every Child Matters*, the Children's Green Paper, September 2003, retrieved 22 July 2008, from www.dfes.gov.uk/everychildmatters

Evans, J. and Davies, B. (2008) 'The poverty of theory: class configurations in the discourse of physical education and health (PEH)', *Physical Education and Sport Pedagogy*, 13(2): 199–213.

Evans, J., Rich, E., Davies, B., and Allwood, R. (2008) *Education, Eating Disorders and Obesity Discourse: Fat Fabrications*. Routledge: London and New York.

Fitzpatrick, T. (2001) *Welfare Theory*, Palgrave: Basingstoke.
Foresight (2005) *Tackling Obesities: Future Choice Projects*, retrieved 27 March 2007, from http://www.foresight.gov.uk/Obesity/Obesity.htm
Foucault, M. (1977) *Discipline and Punish*, London: Peregrine.
Foucault, M. (1979) *Discipline and Punish. The Birth of the Prison*, trans. Alan Sheridan, Harmondsworth: Penguin.
Foucault, M (2003) *Society Must Be Defended*, trans. David Macey, London: Penguin.
Gard and Wright (2005) *The Obesity Epidemic: Science, Morality and Ideology*, London: Routledge.
Government Forum (2008) 'Reducing Youth Offending Generic National Solution', retrieved 27 March 2007, from *http://www.governmentforum365.co.uk/ryogens/*
Howell, P. (2007) 'Foucault, Sexuality, Geography', in J. Crampton and S. Elden (eds) *Space, Knowledge and Power: Foucault and Geography*, Aldershot: Ashgate.
Kelly, M. (2004) 'Racism, nationalism and biopolitics: Foucault's "Society Must Be Defended"', *Contretemps* 4, September: 58–70
Laming, Lord (2003) The Victoria Climbié Inquiry: Report of an inquiry, retrieved 26 June 2008, from http://www.victoria-climbie-inquiry.org.uk/finreport/finreport.htm
Leahy, D. and Harrison, L. (2003) 'Fat laps and fruit straps: childhood obesity, body image, surveillance and education', *NZARE/AARE Conference Abstracts*, NZARE, New Zealand.
Maton, K. (2006) 'On knowledge Structures and Knower Structures', in R. Moore, M. Arnot, J. Beck and H. Daniels (eds) *Knowledge, Power and Educational Reform*, London: Routledge.
Miah, A. and Rich, E. (2008) *The Medicalisation of Cyberspace*. New York: Routledge.
Oliver, K.L., and Lalik, R. (2004) '"The Beauty Walk": Interrogating Whiteness as the Norm for Beauty Within One Schools' Hidden Curriculum', in J. Evans, B. Davies and J. Wright (eds), *Body Knowledge and Control: Studies in the Sociology of Physical Education and Health*, New York: Routledge.
Parton, N. (1998) 'Risk, advanced liberalism and child welfare: The need to rediscover uncertainty and ambiguity', *British Journal of Social Work* 28(1): 5–27.
Penna, S. (2005) 'The Children Act 2004: Child protection and social surveillance', *Journal of Social Welfare and Family Law*, 27(2): 143–157.
Rich, E. and Miah, A. (2006) 'Genetic tests for ability?: Talent identification and the value of an open future', Sport Education and Society, 11(3): 259–273.
Rich, E., and Evans, J. (2007) 'Re-reading voice: Young women, anorexia and performative education', *Junctures*, 9: 39–54.
Seid, P.R. (1989) *Never Too Thin: Why Women Are at War With Their Bodies*, London: Prentice Hall Press.
Shildrick, M. (1997) *Leaky Bodies and Boundaries: Feminism, Postmodernism and (Bio) Ethics*, London: Routledge.
Shilling, C (2008) 'Foreword: Body Pedagogics, Society and Schooling', in J. Evans, E. Rich, B. Davies, and R. Allwood, *Education, Disordered Eating and Obesity Discourse: Fat Fabrications*, London: Routledge.
Shilling, C. and Mellor, P.A. (2007) 'Cultures of embodiment: technology, religion and body pedagogics', *The Sociological Review*, 55(3): 531–549.

12 Disgusting Pedagogies

Deana Leahy

INTRODUCTION

At the present time school based health education is being called upon to respond to yet another crisis. This call to respond to crisis is not new, though the shape of it is. We have been told that we are in the midst of an obesity epidemic, and that schools, in particular health and physical education (HPE), have a role to play in curbing the epidemic. As a result we have witnessed a proliferation of resources, programs and associated teaching strategies directed at cultivating certain bodily practices that are thought to either prevent, or reduce, the risk of being overweight and/or obese. The term biopedagogies, as described by Harwood in Chapter 2 of this collection, encapsulates the very nature and intent of the work that is being done more broadly in schools, as well as in HPE classrooms. In this chapter I bring together and discuss a range of 'biopedagogical' strategies that have been observed across a variety of health education sites.[1] This chapter however offers a new and more nuanced reading and analysis of how various pedagogical devices are deployed and how they might 'do their work' in schools and classrooms. The devices discussed are examples of biopedagogies that are very much directed towards inciting, and building the capacity of, young people to behave in particular ways that align with contemporary governmental imperatives around weight and the body. What becomes evident from the various strategies documented in this chapter is that 'biopedagogies' are complex enactments that invite us back to reconsider previous insights afforded by scholars working in the fields of biopower, governmentality and biopedagogies.

Much of the conceptual terrain around biopedagogies that provides the background to this chapter has been mapped out by Wright in Chapter 1 and Harwood in Chapter 2 in this volume. I am not wanting to rehearse that literature here again; rather I want to add another layer to the analysis. Following Ellsworth (2005) I suggest that to be able to engage with the complexities of biopedagogies and their work, we need to go beyond the field (biopower and governmentality studies) to engage with more experimental and interdisciplinary perspectives to bring new light to understanding and thinking about biopedagogies. Ellsworth (2005: 3–4) believes to grasp how pedagogy functions 'we need concepts and languages that will grasp, without freezing or collapsing, the fluid, continuous, dynamic, multiple, uncertain, non decomposable qualities of experience in the making'. First, I want to suggest that if we are to make sense of how health and physical education classrooms are called on to do 'governmental work' (that is, contribute to shaping the conduct of young people), it is useful to think of the field as a governmental assemblage. This line of thinking follows the recasting of how we might conceive of the project of contemporary governance outlined by Dean (1999) and Rose (2000). Drawing from Deleuze and Guattari's metaphor of assemblages both Rose and Dean offer a very generative way of thinking about contemporary governmental practices. Rose (2000: 322) states that:

> Current control practices manifest, at most, a hesitant, incomplete, fragmentary, contradictory and contested metamorphosis, the abandonment of some old themes, the maintenance of others, the introduction of some new elements, a shift in the role and functioning of others because of their changed places and connections with the 'assemblage' of control.

Similarly, Dean (1999: 29) has alluded to the fragmentary nature of current attempts at governmental regulation and suggests that:

> Practices of government cannot be understood as expressions of a particular principle, as reducible to a particular set of relations, or as referring to a single set of problems or functions. They do not form those types of totalities in which parts are expressions of the whole. Rather they should be approached as composed of heterogeneous elements having diverse historical trajectories, as polymorphous in their internal and external relations, and as bearing upon a multiple and wide range of problems and issues.

Following Rose and Dean's lead here I am going to suggest as I have elsewhere, that school based health education be understood as a governmental assemblage in and of itself with complex linkages and connections to other assemblages (see, for example, Leahy 2007; Leahy and Harrison 2004). This perspective opens up some interesting lines of questioning as to how health education classrooms, and the ensuing biopedagogies, might function in their designated role within the broader governmental assemblage that sets out to prevent, or intervene in, the prevailing obesity crisis. For example, extending on Rose and Dean's analytics above, we might ask: What are the biopedagogies that contribute to the classroom assemblage? How are they assembled? What knowledges are they assembled from? Where are there moments of fragmentation? Where are there contradictions? How do themes or knowledges metamorphise? What do they become? How do new ideas replace or fuse with other ideas? Questions such as these are significant as they invite us to not only engage with the 'how' of government, but also with the messiness that characterizes contemporary projects of governance. This call to think about, and acknowledge, the messiness that characterizes contemporary attempts to govern provides the backdrop to my second point. In considering (bio) pedagogical spaces as assemblages, Ellsworth (2005) and others (for example, Probyn 2004) invite us to consider 'other' forces and dynamics that are at play within classrooms. In many ways the call is to move beyond thinking about biopedagogies as being constituted by expert knowledge alone. By extending this analysis to thinking of other dynamics and affects, we can begin to engage with a more nuanced understanding of how biopedagogies do their governmental work as they come to life in classrooms and work to instill certain dispositions and practices.

HOW HEALTH CLASSROOMS SET OUT TO TACKLE 'THE OBESITY EPIDEMIC'

Given that we discursively find ourselves in the midst of an obesity crisis that is threatening to get worse, it is little wonder that school based health education as a subject area, has been called upon to 'do something'. This 'something' is usually framed within the rhetoric of risk and prevention. The mantra goes, children and young people ARE at risk of becoming overweight/obese AND school based health education is ideally positioned to provide students with relevant attitudes, knowledges and skills that can effectively contribute to reducing this risk. The focus on weight and obesity prevention via the acquisition of attitudes, knowledge and skills is evident across many national and international HPE curriculum and syllabus documents (see Gard and Wright 2005; Burrows and Wright 2004, 2007). It is within this milieu, that we have witnessed a proliferation of biopedagogical strategies designed and adapted to provide students with appropriate learning opportunities to develop and demonstrate the required outcomes. Some of the biopedagogical strategies simply rehearse old themes and approaches as these are called on again by teachers in the preparation of their lesson plans. Some strategies bring together aspects of a variety of approaches from different fields of study. Regardless, a central feature of the development of 'biopedagogical strategies' is a range of expert knowledges drawn from the fields of education and health. As lesson planning continues each biopedagogical strategy is located within a 'scaffold', which means they rub up against each other in an attempt to coherently lead students towards demonstrating the lesson outcomes. Once again approaches to scaffolding are often dependant on prevailing educational expert knowledges. The dominance of expert knowledges here is not surprising, given that many scholars have highlighted the significance of expertise in governing populations (see Dean 1999; Rose 1989). But what is interesting, borrowing from the assemblage metaphor, is how knowledges converge, and morph or even become displaced in what Probyn (2004: 26) refers to as 'the hurly burly of the classroom'. Leahy and Harrison (2004), following Moore and Valverde (2000), have demonstrated how expert knowledges in health education classrooms tend to become hybridized as they are mobilized in classrooms by teachers and students alike. But what is interesting is that expert and hybridized knowledges are only part of the pedagogic assemblage. This chapter seeks to extend on the primacy afforded knowledge in existing analyses, in an attempt to see what other forces and factors are at play in biopedagogical moments.

THE BIOPEDAGOGICAL STRATEGIES OF HEALTH EDUCATION

The ensuing discussion will interrogate a number of biopedagogical strategies that have been, and no doubt are being, utilized in health education classrooms. For the analytical purposes of the chapter, each of these biopedagogical strategies has been 'isolated' for examination. While this does remove the strategy from the broader context of a whole lesson, this approach provides a way to interrogate the minutiae of these strategies.

Assembling Knowledges—Biopedagogic Strategy One

As previously discussed, knowledge is of central importance in a health education classroom. This is not surprising nor new as the field has long been characterized by an emphasis on developing health knowledges (see Lupton 1995). The assumption underpinning a focus on building knowledge is based on the premise that if we have knowledge we can change our behaviour. Although this idea has both been rejected and contested over time and subsequently reconfigured in various policy documents, it still holds a great deal of currency. This emphasis can be observed via analysis of curriculum documents, circulating health education resources, and subsequently many health education classes on a day to day basis. Given the emphasis on knowledge acquisition in health education classrooms, the health education teacher spends a great deal of time developing strategies that create opportunities for students to develop appropriate knowledges (nutritional in the case described later in this chapter). Teachers employ a vast range of strategies to meet this end. Some of those that I have observed include research projects, worksheets, text book tasks and discussion. But I want to suggest however, that knowledge, on its own does not constitute a biopedagogical device, and it is only one aspect of a complex biopedagogical assemblage. This suggestion is not new, and borrows from Rabinow and Rose (2006) in wanting to consider the multivarious elements of biopower. With reference to their work the key nutritional knowledges could be understood as 'knowledge of vital life processes' (p. 215). But as Harwood (this volume) suggests in order to grasp the very nature of biopedagogical work we also need to understand the processes of subjectification. In this case we might ask then how knowledges are folded into the students' understandings of themselves and others[2]. It is this folding action, where knowledge in this case is deliberately mobilized to entice students to understand and relate to themselves in particular ways that gives us the 'bio' of 'biopedagogy'. The following excerpt taken from classroom observational data of a year 10 HPE class highlights the attempt of pedagogical folding in of knowledge, embedding it into how students might understand themselves and their lives. The following exchange comes from an introductory class on the topic. The teacher began:

Ms Murry[3]: Okay today we are going to be looking at nutrition, and I want you to write everything down that you ate yesterday and today already.
Class: General groan.

The teacher's instructions go on to inform students that they will be required to compare what they have eaten with recommended daily intakes and make recommendations to themselves based on what they find out.

The strategy at one level is aimed at developing student understandings of nutrients and the recommended daily intakes as prescribed by the relevant nutritional authority. But the potency of this particular biopedagogical strategy does not reside in the acquisition of knowledge in and of itself. Rather it has more to do with asking students to come to understand themselves and their daily food intake in relation to the nutritional knowledges. In documenting 'everything that they ate yesterday' and then completing a nutritional analysis, the pedagogy is explicitly summonsing students to self monitor, which in turn leads to the expectation that they self regulate food intake (being asked to make recommendations to themselves so that they meet the guidelines).

This actual 'classroom moment' permits us to develop a more intricate understanding as to how governmental and thus biopedagogical imperatives might actually play out. Clearly expert knowledges are central to the outcome of this strategy, but 'success' here, at least in theory, lies with the pedagogical approach that insists that students come to know 'themselves' via their daily intake, and then, where appropriate, make modifications. But I also want to suggest that there is much more going on in this classroom than just the interweaving and folding in of students and expert knowledges. I now turn to discuss some other factors that make up the biopedagogical assemblage.

Assembling Affects—Some More About Biopedagogical Strategy One and then Biopedagogical Strategy Two

In revisiting the initial overview of the strategy by the teacher detailed above, after students received the instructions, the class responded with a 'collective groan'. And although not specified in the audio transcripts of the interview, the groan was accompanied by a range of facial and bodily gestures that suggested a certain level of discomfort and reluctance to record what had been consumed. Although there is much to be said about student responses here, for the purposes of this chapter I want to suggest that the bodily 'affects' generated and sustained throughout the implementation of this particular strategy have significant implications for those of us who are interested in coming to understand governmental and biopedagogical work. This line of analysis follows Tambouko's (2003: 209) suggestion of the need to revisit 'education as a site of intense power relations at play, but [consider it] also as a plane for the production of intense flows of desire and affect'. There are several other writers in education who have also suggested a need to consider the complex interweavings of affect into educational spaces (see, for example, Albrect-Crane and Slack 2007; Probyn 2004; Watkins 2003 and Walkerdine in Chapter 14, this volume). Although their work does not originate from the field of governmentality studies, I would argue that the insights afforded here are significant for future governmental analyses of how biopedagogies are both put to work, and do their work. In many ways when Rose (2000) and Dean (1999) recast the notion of governmentality as an assemblage, they in a sense are asking us to engage with the messiness of the governmental project. To date there have been very few studies that have followed this line. Rather, as I have suggested previously, much of our time and effort has been dedicated to interrogating the role of expertise as it informs and shapes governmental work. This is significant work, however, in order to develop a more nuanced understanding of the complexities at play in pedagogical moments we need to supplement our analyses with other conceptual lens. What might this mean for how we come to understand the operation of biopedagogies? Harwood (this volume) draws on recent theorizations of pedagogy to suggest that biopedagogies are indeed complex phenomena that are 'practices that impart knowledge writ large, occurring at multiple levels across countless domains and sites'. However she also warns that to understand biopedagogies as an enactment of knowledge alone would potentially oversimplify the complexity involved. Ellsworth (1997: 6) offers a way forward in coming to think about pedagogical work as being more than knowledge alone in suggesting that we need to also think of [bio] pedagogy as a 'social relationship [that] is very close in. It gets right in there in your brain, your body, your heart, in your sense of self, of the world, of others, and of possibilities and impossibilities in all those realms'. In a sense Ellsworth (1997) is alluding here to processes of subjectification, the how of pedagogy, as it is developed and deployed to get close in. It is here where thinking about affect becomes valuable as it might be recruited as part of the biopedagogical assemblage. From the above example (and others that follow) we can begin to see how pedagogies are explicitly designed to permeate and creep into students' ways of thinking and being. It is not just about being able to recite nutrients and their effects (that is, expert discourses). The collective groan tells us it is so very much more than that. Bodily responses and affects are very much part of the pedagogical assemblage of health education, and they are indeed potent when recruited to assist health education work towards its governmental imperatives. I want to turn now to provide another example of a biopedagogical strategy that in its attempts to entice young people to eat well and exercise deliberately mobilizes significant bodily affects to instill a particular message about bodies.

Biopedagogical Device Two

The excerpt that follows was an 'activity' that introduced students to the lesson focus 'health problems associated with being unfit'. The teacher posed the question:

> **Ms Hill:**   Okay what is wrong with being unfit?
> **Class:** [all at once] You get fat, look like Homer Simpson, yuk, you
>   could die.
> **Ms Hill:** So well if you don't want to look like Homer it's important to
>   exercise to keep fit.
>
> [Year 10 HPE class]

The strategy being utilized here by the teacher is that of class discussion. The purpose of the discussion is linked to developing students' awareness of some of the health problems associated with being unfit. The very question in and of itself here is interesting, with the teacher asking, 'What is wrong with being unfit?' The assumption is, without question, that being unfit is indeed wrong. This line of enquiry affords only certain replies. And as student responses attest, being unfit is clearly unacceptable. The range of responses includes a mix of knowledges that rely on problematic assumptions that seek to establish a causal relationship between being unfit = getting fat = dying. These assumptions, albeit they are worth challenging in themselves, can be traced to the circulation of expert knowledges relating to heart disease and the associated contributing risk factors. But another reading of this scenario suggests that being unfit = looking like Homer Simpson = yuk. Evident within the class is a degree of disgust, a powerful affect, that doesn't go unheeded as the teacher draws on the example to make her point. Students should not worry about dying, which is what expert knowledges would have us be concerned about, rather, they should be more worried about looking like Homer Simpson. As I observed this classroom interaction, I witnessed the students pull all sorts of faces in response to this, clearly some were repulsed and disgusted at the idea (and some were not paying any attention at all). This biopedagogical strategy does rely on some expert knowledges, but it is the mobilization of disgust that is, I argue, central. As Lupton and Peterson (1996) note, disgust is a powerful mechanism that has long been deliberately deployed in health promotion campaigns in an attempt to change behaviours. Other writers have alluded to the existence of the unhealthy, abject other in health education curriculum documents and practices (see Burrows and Wright 2007; Wright and Dean 2007). The way in which disgust is mobilized here in the classroom provides some insight as to how this disgusting, abject unhealthy other is bought to life in classrooms. And more importantly how such a concept relies on an affective dimension that elicits a bodily response. But what are the consequences of such practices? What might it mean for students who are encouraged to feel disgusted at an obese other? How does that affective experience fold itself into how people understand themselves in relation to their body, and to others' bodies (obese or not)? Several writers (see, for example, Cohen and Johnson 2005; Hancock 2004; Miller 1997) suggest that disgust is accompanied by certain moralising forces, which have significance for the apportioning of a person's worth and blame (for obesity in this case). In addition, disgust does significant governmental work in peda-gogical spaces by mobilizing and interweaving a bodily response that seems to repel and set oneself apart from the obese body.

Disgust is one affect that is actively mobilized in health education class-room spaces. Both students and teachers call on it when responding to cer-tain behaviours, bodies or beliefs. However, it is only one of the affects that are deliberately mobilized within various biopedagogical assemblages, and thus strategies aimed at preventing childhood obesity. This constellation of affects can be exceptionally potent and the following biopedagogical strategy of lunchbox surveillance exemplifies the reliance on certain affects in the classroom.

Biopedagogical Device Three

The pedagogical device of lunchbox surveillance was observed at a profes-sional development program that I attended as part of data collection for my PhD. The device appears to be a popular one and has similarly been documented in other research (see Burrows and Wright 2007). The session rationale was described by the presenter as arising out of the need to curb the alarming rise of childhood obesity. The presenter then went on to say that there was a whole suite of strategies that could be mobilized in an attempt 'to curb the problem'. While there is much to be made of the many suggested strategies and how they might come together in classrooms, for the purpose of this chapter I am going to discuss a strategy loosely titled 'Let's see what we have in our lunchbox'. The strategy calls on teachers to check students' lunch boxes as they sit down to eat. The purpose of this is to reinforce 'good choices' by highlighting them when they are noticed. This might mean that if a student, for example, has a banana in their lunch box, the teacher would make this into a biopedagogical moment. The teacher here could make an explicit mention of the lunchbox contents and perhaps deliver some nutritional knowledge about the particular item. Or it could be a 'biopedagogical' moment that stimulates discussion. The presenter then added that there were other tactics that a teacher might draw from. She explicitly encouraged the use of public praise for 'good ' lunch boxes and the silent treatment for bad lunchboxes. There was mention that if a teacher wanted to communicate that a student had a 'bad' lunchbox they could quietly walk past the offending child and lunchbox and let out a 'tsk tsk' to let it be known to that student that their lunchbox was not acceptable.

There are to be sure many variations of lunchbox surveillance as a device as described above (see, for example, the curriculum resource, *Primary Fight-back*, International Diabetes Institute 2003). The mandate for conducting such strategies gains its support from risk discourses and expert knowledges. But once again from the example above, expert knowledges are not what are being recruited to do governmental work, though they are never far away. Expert knowledges hover in the background and are called upon at various times to highlight, for example, what constitutes a good choice or not. They are very much a part of the assemblage. However, this strategy attests to the significance of utilizing a constellation of affects, including pride, shame and disgust. The intention is–clear. The student should feel embarrassed, and ashamed of their lunchbox. These affects are deliberately recruited via the biopedagogical device in an attempt to entice children to behave in particular ways. We cannot know what the bodily and emotional responses are for those children who are praised or shamed because of their lunchbox contents from this piece of data. On the very surface the intention is that praise will reinforce a positive behaviour so that it continues. For those whose lunchboxes were subjected to a negative teacher response, for example the "tsk tsk-ing" of the teacher, or having to sit and endure their teacher's silence, the very experience is explicitly designed to make the child feel uncomfortable, to shame them into bringing a better lunch box. The message is clear, if they bring a 'good' lunch box they can avoid having to bear the brunt of the bodily discomfort of shame. In addition, the 'good' lunch box may actually become an exemplar that they could then feel proud of.

Disgusting Pedagogies

The three pedagogic devices discussed above, all in varying degrees are designed to bring about behaviour change related to diet and/or activity levels as 'we' attempt to curtail the 'present obesity epidemic'. Whether or not the strategies achieve their objective, we cannot know. Regardless of this concern, biopedagogical strategies that target the body and the self in such ways are powerful. From the data outlined above it becomes clear that expert knowledges contribute significantly to the development, and deployment of biopedagogical strategies. But they are not on their own. Powerful affects are recruited by teachers and students as part of what I would refer to as the pedagogical assemblage. The mobilization of the affects of shame, guilt, pride and disgust alongside expert knowledges provides a different way of conceptualizing the 'how' of biopedagogies, and governmentality more broadly. The potential impact of such practices on young people, how they might come to know and understand themselves, as well as others, requires careful consideration. Admittedly the data discussed here cannot reveal the immediate, nor enduring effects, of what it is to deliberately produce the experience of shame around the body and around food. Nor from this data can we truly know what it might be like for a young person sitting in a classroom, who might be uncomfortable about their body, to experience a collective groan of disgust from their peers directed at a body they might feel they have. One can only imagine. The biopedagogical strategies and resultant assemblages are indeed disgusting for this very reason.

Biopedagogies, as they do their governmental work, rely on a potent assemblage of knowledges and affects. In this case the biopedagogy is set to work when the teacher scaffolds teaching and learning initiatives that both interweave and fold expert knowledges into and onto the body. Actively working to produce affect alongside the expert knowledges permits this folding to take place. Classrooms are indeed complex spaces, made up of a vast assemblage of objects, bodies, curriculum imperatives and pedagogical practices that are connected to broader assemblages. There is much value I suggest in conceptualizing the field as a governmental assemblage and in so doing, considering all of what is going on in that assemblage. Expert risk knowledges are significant, but we need other conceptual tools to take to the study of governmentality if we are to more acutely understand some of the nuances of the governmental project of health education, and I would argue, other pedagogical fields. The various constellations being produced as a result of this crisis are indeed worrying.

NOTES

1. The data discussed were observed as part of a multi site, multi method case study of health education in Victoria. See also Leahy (2007); Leahy and Harrison (2004, 2006).
2. The fold is a Deleuzian concept that was developed as a way of understanding Foucault's later work on subjectification. See Deleuze (1988).
3. All names are pseudonyms.

REFERENCES

Albrect-Crane, C. and Slack, J. (2007) 'Toward a Pedagogy of Affect', in A. Hickey-Moody and P. Malins (eds) *Deleuzian Encounters: Studies in Contemporary Social Issues*, London: Palgrave Macmillan.

182   Deana Leahy

Burrows, L. and Wright, J. (2004) 'The Discursive Production of Childhood, Identity and Health', in J. Evans, B. Davies and J. Wright (eds) *Body Knowledge and Control: Studies in the Sociology of Physical Education and Health*, Routledge: London.

——.(2007) 'Prescribing practices: shaping healthy children in schools', *International Journal of Children's Rights*,15(6): 83–98.

Cohen, W. and Johnson, R. (2005) *Filth, Dirt, Disgust and Modern Life*, Minneapolis: University of Minnesota Press.

Dean, M. (1999) *Governmentality: Power and Rule in Modern Society*, London: Sage.

Deleuze, G. (1988) *Foucault*, London: Athlone.

Ellsworth, E. (2005) *Places of Learning: Media, Architecture, Pedagogy*, New York: Routledge Falmer.

——.(1997) *Teaching Positions: Difference, Pedagogy and the Power of Address*, New York: Teachers College Press.

Gard, M. and Wright, J. (2005) *The Obesity Epidemic: Science, Morality and Ideology*. New York: Routledge.

Hancock, A.M. (2004) *The Politics of Disgust: The Public Identity of the Welfare Queen*, New York: New York University Press.

International Diabetes Institute (2003) *Primary Fightback: Healthy Eating and Physical Activity*, Caulfied, Victoria: International Diabetes Institute.

Leahy, D. (2007) 'School health education and risk messages', a paper presented at *IUHPE World Conference*, Vancouver, Canada, June.

Leahy, D. and Harrison, L. (2004) 'Health and Physical Education and the Production of the 'At Risk Self'', in J. Evans, B. Davies and J. Wright (eds) *Body Knowledge and Control: Studies in the Sociology of Physical Education and Health*, Routledge: London.

——.(2006) 'Producing the 'Unhealthy' Other: School Lunches, Obesity and Governmentality', *Investing in the Future of Every Child: School Meals, Health, Social Capital and Attainment*, Hull, UK: University of Hull.

Lupton, D. (1995) *The Imperative of Health: Public Health and the Regulated Body*, London: Sage.

Lupton, D. and Peterson, A. (1996) *The New Public Health: Health and Self in the Age of Risk*, Sydney: Allen & Unwin.

Miller, W. (1997) *The Anatomy of Disgust*, Cambridge: Harvard University Press.

Moore, D. and Valverde, M. (2000) 'Maidens at risk: Date rape drugs and the formation of hybrid risk knowledges', *Economy and Society*, 29: 514–531.

Probyn, E. (2004) 'Teaching bodies: Affects in the classroom', *Body and Society*, 10: 21–43.

Rose, N. (1998) *Inventing Our Selves: Psychology, Power, and Personhood*, Cambridge: Cambridge University Press.

——.(2000) 'Government and control', *British Journal of Criminology*, 40: 321–39.

Tambouko, M. (2003) 'Interrogating the "emotional turn": Making connections with Foucault and Deleuze', *The European Journal of Psychotherapy, Counselling and Health*, 6: 209–23.

Watkins, M. (2003) *Discipline and Learn: Theorising the Pedagogic Body*, Unpublished Phd Thesis, University of Western Sydney.

Wright, J. and Dean, R. (2007) 'A balancing act—problematising prescriptions about food and weight in school health texts', *Utbildning och Demokrati: tidsskrift foer didaktik och utbildningspolitik*, 16(2): 75–94.

13 The Rise of the Corporate Curriculum

Fatness, Fitness, and Whiteness

Laura Azzarito

INTRODUCTION

In Western societies, educational policies, research, and pedagogies across a range of disciplines are increasingly being driven by 'neoliberal globalism', a neocolonial initiative toward deterritorialization, universalization, and monodimensional standardization (Apple, Kenway, and Singh 2005). While, on one hand, globalizing education espouses and legitimates discourses of difference in increasingly diverse schools, on the other hand, these current trends produce and sustain monocultural and acontextual educational discourses that erase difference (Apple, Kenway, and Singh 2005), and, in turn, homogenize youths' bodies through schooling (Pinar 2004). One form of this homogenization has been large-scale obesity research interventions and preventions in schools (Flores 1995; Pangrazi 2006; Sallis, McKenzie, Alcaraz, Kolody, Faucette, and Hovell 1997).

At the same time, these urgent demands for fitness and health education take place in a time of cultural hybridization, a moment when there is increasing 'difference' across transcendent, virtual borders (Asher 2002). Such advocacy for curricular interventions has paid particular attention to 'diverse' young people because they are believed to be disproportionately affected by the so-called 'obesity epidemic' (Flores, Fuentes-Afflick, Barbot, Carter-Pokras, Claudio, Lara, McLaurin, Pachter, Ramos Gomez, Mendoza, Burciaga Valdez, Villarruel, Zambrana, Greenberg, Weitzman 2007). Increasingly it seems, the obesity epidemic is becoming the 'Other's' problem.

In the context of the so-called global obesity epidemic, the assumptions sustaining discourses about the body, race, health, and fitness warrant further scrutiny. First, the fat body paradoxically coexists with the fabrication of the globally available, fit (slender/muscular) body; it is circumscribed not only by the obesity epidemic discourse, but also by racialized discourses that locate racial / ethnic minority and poor young people as fatter than the white and upper-class. Sustained by new economies, new pedagogies (i.e., internet, media, TV), and health imperatives, the fit body, in opposition to the fat body, represents a desirable, commodified site of transformation for the consumption of globally available symbolic capital. In contrast to the fat body, the fit body symbolizes the disciplined, efficient, and productive body (Azzarito 2007b). The fit body is a transcendent, healthy body constructed upon gendered, white ideals (Seid 1989), and pedagogized through the media and the emergence of the medical, health, and fitness alliance manifest in alarmist discourses of the world-wide obesity epidemic.

Another dominant assumption that underpins health imperatives is the notion that fitness and low-fat dieting are beneficial and necessary for 'everyone.' Whites are reported as the healthiest and fittest, with no attention paid to the ways young people's cultural experiences, history, and locations shape their physicality. The intangible, but omnipresent mechanism of whiteness denies non-white young people the prerogative to understand relevant meanings constructed around their physicality, and to engage in, or learn about, alternative and more culturally relevant body knowledge. Whiteness, as Lee (2005: 4) notes, is 'invisible and ubiquitous in defining "American-ness"'. The colour-blindness of new monocultural fitness and health crusades in school physical education panopticizes non-whites, the populations most at risk for fatness, as visibly different, abnormal, unhealthy and lazy; and it leaves the underlying assumptions of whiteness unexamined. What is required are approaches that dismiss the biological 'marking' of ethnicity and embrace an interdisciplinary approach to understanding the etiology of persistent health inequalities among different ethnic groups. Such an approach suggests the need, and provides the means, to investigate the ways in which large-scale fitness and dieting interventions in schools implicitly work to colonize minority young people's physicality to homogenous, monocultural, white conceptions of the 'fit, slim body.'

Campaigns against fatness concurrently contribute to the rise of 'business-minded' schooling reform, academic analogues to 'the bottom line (i.e., profit)' with 'tendencies toward cultural homogenization' (Pinar 2004: 94), and the rise of the corporate curriculum. The top-down approach of the corporate curriculum model, with its emphasis on test scores and standardization, is implicated in the regulation of race and the social body. With the rise of business-minded school reform, whiteness fluidly operates through neocolonial practices of categorizing, naming and classifying the body (i.e., BMIs) to alleviate the social anxieties of the obesity crisis. This chapter therefore is concerned with the emergence of school-based health and fitness research interventions and academic conversations about health and fitness specifically targeting minority young people.

While I do not discount researchers' good intentions and urgency in developing school-based research approaches to enhancing young people's health, the lack of cultural and historical conversations about the links among schooling, health, culture, and ethnicity in the planning and reporting of this research is worrisome. In this chapter, my critical analysis of the dominant discourses of fitness, healthism, and race/ethnicity informing school-based research, school health practices, and researchers' adoption of language, as well as the ways these discourses construct non-white young people, unfolds in several points. First, I contend that emerging school interventions, supposedly educationally based, are narrowly built upon the medicalization of young people's bodies, disavowing a socio-historical understanding of the construction of health and fitness discourses as embedded in whiteness, and implicitly function as a 'blaming the victim' approach. Second, complicit with neoliberal political trends, the development and implementation of large-scale fitness and health interventions in schools specifically targeting non-white young people have the potential to recreate and/or reinforce racialized categories by reclaiming race as a biological category through fatness. Third, although there have been some efforts to develop interventions using multicultural approaches, from a postcolonial perspective, these 'culturally relevant' fitness/dieting approaches tend to rely on assimilating the bodies of young people from different ethnic backgrounds to whiteness. I conclude this chapter by arguing for the necessity to decolonize young people's bodies by shifting educational, cultural, and political efforts toward understanding how young people make sense of their bodies in relation to health and participation in physical activity.

WHITENING FAT BODIES: 'ONE SIZE FITS ALL'!

Fitness, Health, and Fat-Phobia: A 'White Thing'?

> Ideas and categories from the medical community about the body continue to shape cultural aspiration, national character, immigration barriers and population policy.
>
> (Anderson 2003: 258)

In fitness and health-based corporate curricula, the lack of attention to cultural differences and the historical contingencies of young people's bodies threatens to engulf and re-colonize minority physicality. It is through the monocultural and ahistorical language of discourses of fatness and fitness in schools that young people's bodies, in subtle ways, are pedagogized to white ideals of the body. For instance, according to doctors, health advocates, and politicians, schools represent ideal sites for developing and implementing large-scale interventions aimed at regulating young people's diets and levels of physical activity. Like others (Pangrazi 2006; Warren, Henry, Lightowler, Bradshaw, and Perwaiz 2003), Fitzgibbon, Stolley, Shiffer, Van Horn, KauferChristoffel and Dyer (2006: 1616) assert that the school is 'an excellent setting for the promotion of healthy eating and activity among children'. The argument is as follows: To change children's diet- and physical activity-related behavior, first, school 'physical education programs that emphasize and model learning of daily activities for personal fitness' should be promoted; second, 'healthy choices'—low-fat milk, vegetables, and fruit—should be provided in school cafeterias. With these aims, educators, health promoters, and researchers have started to advocate for physical education, health, and fitness interventions that have been demonstrated as effective in improving children's health-related physical fitness in predominantly white schools (e.g., *Sport, Play, and Active Recreation for Kids* [SPARK]) in more ethnically and socio-economically diverse schools (Sallis et al. 1997), specifically targeting minority children (Flores et al. 2007).

While the common point of these interventions targeting minority populations centres on increasing fitness exercise and reducing Body Mass Index (BMI) through dieting, the monocultural assumptions of these schooling interventions deny the hidden historical construction of fitness and dieting practices as a 'white thing.' What remains invisible in researchers' assumptions, approaches, and conversations about non-white young people and health is the way the Anglo-American children's body size and shape are constructed as the norm, hierarchically superior to those of minorities, and the way dieting, fitness practices, and fat-phobic values are rooted historically in Anglo-American culture. Without excavating the relationship between the social construction of racialized discourses of fatness and fitness, 'whiteness then becomes acontextual and all encompassing, the unspoken, taken-for-granted way of being human' (Cuomo and Hall 1999: 73).

Briefly considering health and fitness initiatives of the past few decades can help us contextualize the contemporary 'urgency' around fighting fatness in schools, as well as the particular focus on the minority body. Only a few decades ago, 'Shape up America!' was a central cultural, economic, and political message, rooted, indeed, in anti-fat and anti-brown rhetoric (Azzarito 2007a). Politicians' and health advocates' discourses of 'Shape up America!' emerged during the American public school reform period of the 1960s, a time that Pinar (2004) describes as marking the genesis of today's standards-driven, business-minded education for curriculum consumers. Pinar (2004: 7) argues that in this regressive time for education, 'the genesis of our nightmare was [not only] gendered, it was profoundly racialized as well'. During this period, promoting fitness in the school gym played a crucial role in shaping up young people, especially young boys, who were becoming 'too soft.' Implicated in the political and militaristic agenda of the Cold War, 'Shape up America' aimed to cure growing fatness and restore fitness among youth. Fit bodies symbolized boys' manliness and strength through the glorification of athleticism and physical fitness. The President's Council on Physical Fitness in this era launched national fitness testing (later the President's Challenge), which reinforced gendered and racialized norms of the body (Azzarito 2007a).

While for boys, these fitness crusades in schools championed strength, toughness, and courage versus softness, serving as a mechanism to 'redeem manhood' (Pinar 2004: 86), for girls, fitness and dieting signified the possibility of achieving the ideal slender, white body. During this period, according to Seid (1989), the so-called 'Age of Caloric Anxiety,' Americans waged a 'war against fatness'; their obsession with burning calories and dieting responded to, contributed to, and built upon the cultural 'myth of slenderness,' and as Seid (1989: 103) points out, 'Body weight was becoming American's most important measure, a way to gauge health, beauty, and character'. The myth of slenderness, then, inevitably produced not only an obsession with fatness, but also prejudice against it. For instance, as Seid (1989: 159) describes, in this historical moment, fatness was viewed as a 'socially deviant form of physical disability. . . . [I]t was perceived as disgusting, and so those who suffered from it'. By the 1970s, the commodified and consumer-oriented dream of self-transformation promised the achievement of beauty, happiness, and vitality through fitness and dieting practices.

Such fat-phobic concerns about the body, the result of 'social and scientific reforms' of the 1950s, also enforced norms of whiteness. The healthy diet advertised and strongly suggested by doctors centered on vegetables, fruit, and low-fat milk products. While these food products were especially fashionable among the educated white upper class at the time, complex carbohydrates (i.e., bread, potatoes, rice) were medicalized as unhealthy foods and became 'the verboten foods of the period, with the stigma of being fattening added to the stigma of being lower-class' (Seid 1989: 130). This popular diet was racialized in the sense that not only was it was a fad among the white upper class, but it also functioned as a mechanism of assimilation of minorities to white America. As Chamberlain (2001: 101) contends, 'To promote better health, Americanization programs taught Mexican American mothers to substitute white bread for tortillas, green lettuce for frijoles, and boiled meat for fried meat'. Dieting practices circulating among white, upper-middle-class culture, and medicalized as healthy for poor Mexican Americans, concurred with fitness crusades that were launched inside and outside of schools to shape up the young generation (Pinar 2004).

In a context in which the notion of fatness as a disease was sustained, produced, and reinforced by doctors who had 'a professional and economic stake in keeping bodies slim enough to pursue the America dream,' fat, dark bodies represented 'the ultimate American nightmare' (Chamberlain 2001: 92). Fat was distinctly un-American. The provocative narrative of Zeta Acosta, *The Autobiography of a Brown Buffalo*, discloses the ways political, economic, and cultural discourses of fitness, health, and medicalization of the body were racialized, complicit with white America (Azzarito 2007a). Acosta found himself constantly embattled against a society that cast him as a 'greaser' and 'fat' or a 'spoiled identity,' by refusing to conform to white diets, drink low-fat milk, and eat bland food to lose weight. His resistance to doctors and diets not only represented resistance to White America, but was also a source of the intimate, lifelong conflict he embodied in a fat-phobic and racist American context. Acosta's renaming himself as Fat Brown Buffalo signified his negotiation of discrimination against his fatness and discrimination against his darker skin colour, a sense of isolation and disconnection from white America. Acosta's refusal to conform to fitness and health norms represented a complicated, inconsistent, and conflictual personal, cultural, and political issue.

While it is important to recognize the historical, political, and social specificity of Acosta's autobiography, it is arguable that by disavowing history and culture, the contemporary rise of the corporate curriculum through new fitness crusades (i.e., large, school-based fitness and dieting interventions) tacitly functions as a neocolonial initiative to reinforce whiteness. Without historical and social awareness, the language adopted by researchers developing health-fitness school-based interventions functions as a 'blaming the victim' discourse, maintaining whiteness as invisible. Racialized discourses are produced when researchers attribute the lack of significant results of diet and physical activity research intervention in decreasing BMI to the low acculturation of Latino parents, the difficulty in altering high-fat Latino diets, and the unhealthy environments where they live, contexts that promote 'inactivity and the consumption of highly caloric and palatable foods' (Fitzgibbon et al. 2006: 1623).

Discourses of whiteness are implicitly sustained by researchers' adoption of stereotypical, racialized discourses that discount historical constructions of health, diet, and the body. Researchers' use of current evidence of the health disparities by race/ethnicity and social class to locate minorities as an economic and social burden on the national economy is the basis for a racialized discourse of 'blaming the victim.' As Barlow and the Expert Committee of *Pediatrics* (2007) acknowledge, individuals' ethnic cultural values and historical traditions are crucial in shaping their identities and sense of health, and thus it is important that clinicians not disavow these values. In this report, the authors suggest that clinicians tailor obesity health-related recommendations to the individuals and communities they serve: for example, they should not advise Mexican Americans to change a traditional Mexican diet; nor should a Mexican American diet be stigmatized as 'bad' or 'unhealthy.' Rather, clinicians should legitimate culturally relevant diets emphasizing, at the same time, healthy aspects of or healthy compromises within ethnic diets. Importantly, in poor communities, community providers should offer low-cost, healthy foods that are the most consistent with the community members' culture. As Thomas (2006: 790) suggests, a 'one size fits all approach' to research on youth obesity prevention and intervention school programs is not relevant to certain ethnic groups.

Naturalizing the Other's Fatness and Lack of Fitness

> Panicky whiteness's vilification of non-white—blacks and Latinos in particular—holds very specific consequences. The power of whiteness simply cannot be separated from its control of the economy.
>
> (Kincheloe and Steinberg 2002: 224).

Just as academic failure among minorities historically has been rationalized as either a cultural deficit or a genetic deviance measurable via standardized achievement tests (McCarthy 1990: 8), in Western societies today, the health and fitness status of fat minority youths is rearticulated as a lack of the normative physical capital necessary to become fit, productive, and efficient citizens. In the United States, as well as in Europe and Australia, mainstream research based on positivist, empiricist approaches, involving quantification, and measurement and the comparison against white standards has a long history of stabilizing racialized discourses of the 'deviance' of disadvantaged non-white groups (Anderson 2003). For instance, the use of quantitative measures of intelligence, such as the IQ test that reflects the 'normative performance of middle-class white males,' exemplifies racist schooling practices (McCarthy 1990: 18).

Naturalizing the Other's body objectifies its fatness and lack of fitness because, according to Asher (2005: 1083), it is 'the colonizing gaze of the white man that objectifies the black man'. For example, in claiming the urgent need for large fitness and health interventions in schools, the taken-for-granted assumption of targeting minorities relies on the notion that non-white youths are fat or likely to become fat, are disadvantaged or 'deviate' from the norm, and thus constitute a burden to the nation. Dangerously, through these scientific quantifications and classifications of the body (i.e., fatness and fitness), race is reclaimed as a 'biological marker.' As such, school curriculum initiatives that subject minority bodies to skinfold measurements, BMI classification, and physical activity quantifications aim to measure physical capital disadvantage or deviance from the normative, white performance.

If they are not culturally sensitive, the language researchers use in reporting on school-based interventions, specifically targeting minorities' obesity issues, produces and reinforces racialized discourses of health that settle racialized categories of the body. For instance, in a report on a recent school intervention, the research team's interpretation of their results classifies and homogenizes minority children, racializing discourses of fatness: 'Mexican-American children in this sample were shown to be *deficient* in many variables thought to be important for physical activity, so this group is in need of targeted interventions to help them overcome these disadvantages' (Morgan, McKenzie, Sallis, Broyles, Zive, and Nader 2003: 298). The authors' analysis of the bodies of the minority children in the study centers on their greater total skinfold thickness, lower physical self-perception, lower enjoyment of physical activity, and greater contextual barriers, such as poor neighborhood safety and fewer community resources and facilities. In this comparison, adequate physical activity, good health, and safe environments become racialized norms equated with whiteness, where differences in contexts, resources, attitudes, and habits mark the first group as 'deficient.' If racialized norms are to be seriously challenged, then researchers' conversations should emphasize the importance of access and opportunities for *all* young people's participation in physical activity and should insist on politicians' and community and school authorities' advocating for the establishment and maintenance of safe parks, school physical activity facilities, and recreation centers that young people, especially young people who live in poor communities, can access.

Two other interventions (Caballero, Clay, Davis, Ethelbah, Holy Rock, Lohman, T., Norman, Story, Stone, Stephenson and Stevens 2003; Gittelsohn, Evans, Helitzer, Anliker, Story, Metcalfe, Davis, and Iron Cloud 1998), which tested and quantified non-white young people's bodies, also re-constructed these specific ethnic populations as deviant or deficient from the normative white. The first was a large school-based study targeting six different Native American communities, in which researchers aimed to develop and test a fitness and dieting intervention 'to establish healthy lifestyle behaviour' that would reduce obesity or the risk of obesity among Native American children during their adulthood (Gittelsohn et al. 1998). The second (Caballero et al. 2003) focused on dietary intake change, increased fitness exercise, and family involvement to reduce the percentage of body fat among Native American children. The problem with such quantitative health and fitness interventions is that they define ethnic groups as homogeneous, racialized groups, an assumption Henderson and Ainsworth (2001: 20) describe as 'fallacies of homogeneity and monolithic identity'. Targeting specific non-white populations dangerously and implicitly locates minority populations as the Other, and reclaims ethnicity as a genetic category. Despite scientific agreement about the unclear etiology of obesity, reports in the United States and the United Kingdom have consistently argued that minorities' high risk of obesity and physical inactivity compared to whites legitimates schooling interventions; such interventions ultimately work to homogenize ethnic groups, and naturalize race and its link to fatness. It conceals the heterogeneity of ethnic groups and ignores the scientific data establishing that race itself does not exist biologically; that is, it is an empty scientific category, as race does not have general genetic markers (Cuomo and Hall 1999: 83). Indeed, as Nazroo (2003: 277) argues in his discussion of ethnic inequalities in health, 'given the growing empirical and theoretical sophistication of work on ethnic inequalities in health, it is worrying that crude explanations based on cultural stereotypes and claims of genetic difference persist'.

Schools, as institutional sites crucial to managing and regulating the body, have become the place in and through which the social body is not only refabricated, but also racialized to healthy, fit, efficient, productive, and white norms (McCarthy 1990). While the deployment of biopower in Western capitalist societies regulates the social body by optimizing its aptitudes, economic forces, and productivity, at the same time, biopower acts to maintain social racialized hierarchization by guaranteeing the effect of hegemonic dominant discourses of the body. To discipline individuals to 'normalcy,' regulatory mechanisms over the social body work to qualify, measure, and categorize by creating the need for biomedical preventions and interventions as corrective or curative regimes for individuals' behaviors. As mechanisms of biopower, fitness and low-fat dietary practices in schools rely on the implicit notion that minorities are more likely to become fat and less productive in globalized Western societies; they therefore are portrayed as a burden not only on single nations, but also on the world, and as inferior to the 'normalcy' of more fit, healthy, and productive white populations.

Multiculturalism, Colour-Blindness, and the 'Other's' Fatness

> Framed thus, by the White man's gaze, multicultural education does not, ultimately, shake the patriarchal foundations of 'the master's house', much less dismantle them.
>
> (Asher 2007: 75)

In this last section, I suggest that researchers use caution when adopting multiculturalism in fitness and health school-based interventions because, from a postcolonial theoretical view, multiculturalism works as an assimilationist approach, employing colour-blind practices that leave whiteness unexamined. Such approaches preclude possibilities for researchers to theorize the ways young people make sense of, construct, and re-construct their physicality as they negotiate globalized discourses of healthism, fitness, and the medicalization of the body. Multicultural fitness and health enterprises in schools legitimate the Other, but through assimilationist efforts to fix the poor, dark, fat body to white ideals.

Several recent health-fitness interventions in American schools have employed multiculturalism as a strategy for improving the health of ethnic minority students. Despite the projects' claims to cultural sensitivity, the underlying, implicit focus of these interventions has been to acculturate participants (i.e., minority youths) to 'appropriate' healthy and physically active lifestyles. *Dance for Health* (Flores 1995), *Hip-hop for Health* (Fitzgibbon et al. 2006), and the Pathways physical activity intervention for Native American children (Caballero et al. 2003), all claimed to offer culturally relevant physical activities for young people, and all shared a similar learning focus: minorities' adoption of 'correct' attitudes toward physical fitness and health, as demonstrated by improved fitness levels and reduced BMI. For instance, *Dance for Health* (Flores 1995) was a school-based, aerobic-exercise intervention, developed and implemented for low-income African American and Latino adolescents, that used hip-hop music as a 'culturally appropriate dance' approach to reducing body weight. In this program, dance routines were developed to appeal to girls and boys of both ethnic groups; however, the curriculum required minimal skills for hip-hop dance, and the physical educational aspects of hip-hop as historically and culturally relevant music and dance were omitted from the curriculum. Thus, the claim that *Dance for Health* incorporated a multicultural approach is misleading, as educational learning outcomes were neither taken into account nor included. By contrast, improving fitness and reducing weight among groups of minority youth was the single, narrow purpose of this normalizing curricular intervention.

With its similar, but more explicit focus on weight control/reduction and fitness, Fitzgibbon et al.'s (2006: 1617) intervention, *Hip-Hop to Health Jr.*, argued for a culturally relevant approach in order to 'take these young children off the trajectory toward obesity as they grew'. Likewise, the multicultural approach of Gittelsohn et al.'s (1998: 251) school-based research was to prevent obesity in six different Native American nations in an effort 'to establish healthy lifestyle behaviour' during childhood. By adding aspects of the Other (American Indian games) to a health-related physical education model framed within the dominant culture, as in Caballero et al.'s (2003) research, this melting pot approach maintained a colour-blind, assimilationist position in relation to the dominant white discourse, which emphasizes 'difference' in efforts to develop 'sameness.'

From a postcolonial view, multiculturalism's focus on 'difference,' its emphasis on acknowledging and celebrating diversity (Pinar, Reynolds, Slattery and Taubman 1996), works as a form of regulation and discipline to the dominant norm, discourses of 'sameness.' Whereas multiculturalism puts effort into making visible the experiences of the Other, multicultural education maintains a dominant culture. This means that whiteness remains at the center, in opposition to the Other's cultures, which occupy positions marginal to the mainstream. The embedded message of multiculturalism, 'we are different but we are all the same' (McCarthy 1990: 52), implicitly maintains a colour-blind orientation that sets back the socio-educational, economic, and racial struggle needed to pursue equality. It falls short of producing authentic, cultural curricular engagement with the interrogation of difference, whiteness, and Othering processes.

In postcolonial terms, multiculturalism is undermined by the neocolonial initiative embedded in its assumptions, by its tendency to treat minority cultures as exotic and monolithic, and thus, again, as different from the dominant, more 'civilized' one. According to Pinar et al. (1996: 324), the curricular interest of multiculturalism is 'the development of competence for the public sphere, i.e. white mainstream culture'. In our globalizing society, while a fit body signifies efficiency, productivity, and beauty ideals, a fat or 'bad' body represents laziness, gluttony, and lack of control (Evans, Rich, and Davies 2004). Despite the unclear etiology of the high risks of obesity among minority youths and adults, representations of minority cultures in discourses of obesity that emphasize poor Latinos', Native Americans', or Blacks' lack of physical activity and consumption of high-fat foods paradoxically reinforce stereotypical views.

Rethinking the relationship between young people's cultures and their physicality and health demands that 'a multicultural pedagogy begins with the transformation of the self, not just the Other' (Asher 2007: 67).

Decolonizing girls and boys from minority ethnic and cultural backgrounds demands that researchers who work with, are committed to, and develop school curricula for youth recognize young people's identities as fluid, with non-homogeneous, inconsistent identifications. It demands that researchers, educators, and clinicians adopt multicultural pedagogies and curricular practices that do not simply assimilate or reproduce stereotypes of the Other's fatness, but rather, that engage us in a cultural and political relationship with Others and fatness in order to excavate underlying racist and classist discourses about the body. As Cuomo and Hall (1999: 85) suggest, the multicultural attempt to deal with 'difference' without seriously challenging white, middle-class privilege, simply remains a dangerous 'racialized act'.

CONCLUSION

Contemporary dominant discourses of health and fitness strip young people's right to make sense of their physicality through a holistic education of the body; and function to dislodge young people from their sense of the self and the constitution of their physicality as it is formed by their upbringing, experiences, and backgrounds. A review of obesity prevention programs for children and youth suggests that the results are 'mixed and modest' (Doak, Visscher, Renders and Seidell 2006: 112). This lack of consistent and successful research outcomes in attempts to 'shape up' minority youth could be explained by young people's negotiations of, resistance to, and rebellion against these disciplining practices of the body. It is possible that young people resist and negotiate what they experience as regulation, discipline, and normalization of their bodies because the normalizing practices of diet and fitness interventions and preventions diverge from their physicality.

At its worst, the rise of the corporate curriculum aims to alleviate the economic burden of unhealthy, unfit, predominantly non-white people on national health costs by reproducing a neocolonial discourse of 'blaming the victim.' At its best, the corporate curriculum allows for the redemption of white guilt through recognizing 'difference.' The comfort of white privilege transforms into discomfort in light of health disparities and lack of access and opportunities to physically active lifestyles among non-white people. In response to corporate demands for an efficient, productive, and fit social body, white guilt is likely to result in moral obligation, a taking of collective responsibility to address injustice (Zack 1999). Researchers, health advocates, clinicians, and educators should move a little further and realize that in western societies, health trends are the result of historical colonialism and institutionalized racism. Unfortunately, a lack of cultural analysis and white self-examination, and the resulting stigmatization of the Other (i.e., fat, dark skin), leave school-based interventions to proliferate as a contemporary whitening project.

What we know about young people's physicality and the complex ways they negotiate cultures, history, and discourses of fatness, health, and fitness is still very limited. The medical-scientific appropriation of schooling through fitness and low-fat dietary interventions does not offer an in-depth understanding of the ways young people make sense of and experience their bodies and health. Nor has the medicalization of schooling fatness/fitness produced significant results. With this chapter, I argue for the need to decolonize young people's bodies by opening up conversations about the body, fatness, health, race, class, and gender. If we are to seriously tackle young people's obesity and health-related problems, young people's stories about their body-health experiences, knowledge, and understandings must be listened to. Public health researchers' use of monolithic approaches to understanding and promoting fitness and health stifles the ways young people's fluid, conflictual, and multiple identities inform the meanings they attach to physical activity and health.

Research efforts that take into account the ways history, culture, and race/ethnicity identity formation shape young people's physicality and the complex ways they negotiate globalized trends should be promoted and valued. Researchers who are invested in improving young people's health and maximizing their lifetime physicality development must be aware of the cultural dominance of whiteness, and engage in self-examination to understand 'racial differences,' not in opposition, but in relation to their own. If educators', researchers', and clinicians' awareness and recognition of the historical, institutional, and social aspects influencing individuals' obesity issues can be incorporated into our research agendas, the openness to reflection about race, culture, and identity might open doors to alternative understandings of how young people make sense of their physicality in relation to obesity issues. I conclude this chapter by echoing James's (2003: 189) call for a reassessment of priorities in researching minorities' health and physical activity engagement: 'The elimination of health disparities—the magnificently democratic goal of Healthy People 2010—cannot be achieved without first *undoing racism*'.

REFERENCES

Anderson, W. (2003) *The Cultivation of Whiteness: Science, Health, and Racial Destiny in Australia*, New York: Basic Books.

Apple, M.W., Kenway, J. and Singh, M. (2005) *Globalizing Education: Policies, Pedagogies, and Politics.* New York: Peter Lang.

Asher, N. (2002) '(En)gendering a hybrid consciousness', *Journal of Curriculum Theorizing*, 18: 81–92.

———.(2005) 'At the interstices: Engaging postcolonial and feminist perspectives for a multicultural education pedagogy in the South', *Teachers College Record*, 107: 1079–106.

———.(2007) 'Made in the (Multicultural) U.S.A.: Unpacking tensions of race, culture, gender, and sexuality in education', *Educational Researcher*, 36: 65–73.

Azzarito, L. (2007a) '"Shape up America!": Understanding fatness as a curriculum project', *Journal of the American Association for the Advancement of Curriculum Studies*, 3: 1–27.

——.(2007b) '"Llegar hasta el final" en educacion fisica: Observando la 'nueva condicion' de la juventud en nuestra era global', in P.P. Sampol, F.J. Ponseti Verdaguer, P.A. Borras Rotger, and J. Vital Conti (eds) *Educacion fisica en el single XXI. Nuevas perspectives nuevos retos [Physucal Education in XXI Century: a new perspective]*, Palma, Spain: Tecfa Group.

Barlow, S.E. and the Expert Committee (2007) 'Expert committee recommendations regarding the prevention, assessment, and treatment of child and adolescent overweight and obesity: Summary report', *Pediatrics*, 120: 164–92.

Caballero, B., Clay, T., Davis, S. M., Ethelbah, B., Holy Rock, B., Lohman, T., Norman, J., Story, M., Stone, E.J., Stephenson, L. and Stevens J. (2003) 'Pathways: a school-based, randomized controlled trial for the prevention of obesity in American Indian schoolchildren', *American Journal Clinical Nutrition*, 78: 1030–8.

Chamberlain, M. (2001) 'Oscar Zeta Acosta's autobiography of a Brown Buffalo: A fat man's recipe for Chicano revolution', in J.E. Braziel and K. LeBesco (eds) *Bodies out of Bounds: Fatness and Transgression*, Berkeley: University of California Press.

Cuomo, C.J. and Hall, K.Q. (1999) 'White Ideas', in C.J. Cuomo, and K.Q. Hall (eds) *Whiteness: Feminist Philosophical Reflections*, Lanham, MA: Rowman and Littlefield.

Doak, C.M., Visscher, T.L.S., Renders, C.M. and Seidell, J.C. (2006) 'The prevention of overweight and obesity in children and adolescents: A review of interventions and programmes', *Obesity Reviews*, 7: 11–136.

Evans, J., Rich, E. and Davies, B. (2004) 'The emperor's new clothes: fat, thin, and overweight. The social fabrication of risk and ill health', *Journal of Teaching in Physical Education*, 23: 372–91.

Fitzgibbon, M.L., Stolley, M.R., Shiffer, L., Van Horn, L., KauferChristoffel, L. and Dyer, A. (2006) 'Hip-Hop to Health Jr. for Latino preschool children', *Obesity*, 14: 1616–25.

Flores, G., Fuentes-Afflick, E., Barbot, O., Carter-Pokras, O., Claudio, L., Lara, M., McLaurin, J.A., Pachter, L., Ramos Gomez, F., Mendoza, F., Burciaga Valdez, R.B., Villarruel, A.M., Zambrana, R.E., Greenberg, R. and Weitzman, M. (2007) 'The health of Latino children: urgent priorities, unanswered questions, and a research agenda', *The Journal of the American Medical Association*, 288: 82–90.

Flores, R. (1995) 'Dance for health: improving fitness in African American and Hispanic adolescents', *Public Health Report*, 110: 189–93.

Gittelsohn, J., Evans, M., Helitzer, D., Anliker, J., Story, M., Metcalfe, L., Davis, S. and Iron Cloud, P. (1998) 'Formative research in a school-based obesity prevention for Native American school children (Pathways)', *Health Education Research*, 13: 251–65.

Henderson, K. and Ainsworth, B.E. (2001) 'Researching leisure and physical activity with women of colour: issues and emerging questions', *Leisure Sciences*, 23: 21–34.

James, S.A. (2003) 'Confronting the moral economy of US racial/ethnic health disparities', *American Journal of Public Health*, 93: 189.

Kincheloe, J.L., and Steinberg, S.R. (2002) *Changing Multiculturalism*, Philadelphia: Open University Press.

Lee, S.J. (2005) *Up Against Whiteness: Race,School, and Immigrant Youth*, New York: Teachers College Press.

McCarthy, C. (1990) *Race and Curriculum: Social Inequality and the Theories and Politics of Difference in Contemporary Research on Schooling*, London: The Falmer Press.

Morgan, C.F., McKenzie, T.L., Sallis, J.F., Broyles, S.L., Zive, M.M. and Nader, P.R. (2003) 'Personal, social, and environmental correlates of physical activity in a bi-ethnic sample of adolescents', *Pediatric Exercise Science*, 15: 288–301.

Nazroo, J.Y. (2003) 'The structuring of ethnic inequalities in health: Economic position, racial discrimination, and racism', *American Journal of Public Health*, 93: 277–84.

Pangrazi, R.P. (2006) 'Gopher sport: "creating a wellness policy". Active and healthy schools'. A paper presented at the *American Alliance for Health, Physical Education, Recreation and Dance*, Salt Lake City, Utah.

Pinar, W.F. (2004) *What is Curriculum Theory?* London: Lawrence Erlbaum.

Pinar, W.F., Reynolds, W.M., Slattery, P. and Taubman, P.M. (1996) *Understanding Curriculum*, New York: Peter Lang.

Sallis, J.F., McKenzie, T.L., Alcaraz, J.E., Kolody, B. Faucette, N. and Hovell, M.F. (1997) 'The effects of a 2-year physical education program (SPARK) on physical activity and fitness in elementary school students', *American Journal of Public Health*, 87: 1328–34.

Sallis, J.F., McKenzie, T.L., Conway, T.L., Elder, J.P., Prochaska, J.J., Brown, M., Zive, M.M., Marshall, S.J. and Alcaraz, J.E. (2003) 'Environmental interventions for eating and physical activity: a randomized controlled trial in middle schools', *American Journal of Preventive Medicine*, 24: 209–17.

Seid, P.R. (1989) *Never Too Thin: Why Women are at War with their Bodies*, London: Prentice Hall.

Thomas, H. (2006) 'Obesity prevention programs for children and youth: why are their results so modest?' *Health Education Research*, 21: 783–95.

Warren, J.M., Henry, C.J.K., Lightowler, H.J., Bradshaw, S.M. and Perwaiz, S. (2003) 'Evaluation of a pilot school programme aimed at the prevention of obesity in children', *Health Promotion International*, 18: 287–96.

Zack, N. (1999) 'The King of Whiteness', in C.J. Cuomo, and K.Q. Hall (eds) *Whiteness: Feminist Philosophical Reflections*, Lanham, MA: Rowman and Littlefield.

Part III

Commentary

14 Biopedagogies and Beyond

Valerie Walkerdine

In commenting on this important selection of papers, my aim is to raise issues so as to stimulate discussion, in order, hopefully, to take some of the discussion forward. In doing this, I will reflect on issues raised for me by some of the papers and add points from my own research if, and when, these seem useful.

There is no doubt that the papers collected in this volume offer an important approach to the study of the pedagogization of weight and obesity. I want to begin by thinking about the thoughtful chapter by Michael Gard in which he situates his own and Jan Wright's (2005) previous book, *The Obesity Epidemic: Science, Morality and Ideology*. In particular, the central importance of the paper for me is that it erodes our sense of certainties about the practice of critique. We are used, as many papers in this volume do and I have done myself, to cite a number of critical theorists, Foucault and Deleuze for example, to establish out credentials, to stake out a position from which we speak. But, as Gard makes clear, we have not paid enough attention to how our work is received both academically and popularly. To find, as Gard found, that no-one in the obesity mainstream was taking notice of their work is one thing, but then to discover that the critique was taken up by groups differently opposed to the obesity mainstream, by Right- wing libertarians on the one hand and fat pride activists, on the other, is something of a shock. This suggests that we need to understand the production and utilisation of knowledge in the present in a much more complex way than we are used to doing, as well as understanding the role of critique and indeed political and theoretical intervention.

In the present political conjuncture, we find single issue politics, new alliances beyond left and right. This suggests that traditional modes of opposition and critique, often directed at a government, for example, simply do not even vaguely match the complexity of the current political situation. I am reminded both of the centrality of chaos and complexity to some developments in attempts to understand processes of globalisation (see Urry 2003) and work which suggests that we simply cannot predict the ways in which rhizomatic flows will work (Deleuze and Guattari 2004) or creation happen (Bergson 1911). The engagement with these approaches by social and cultural theorists can be understood as an attempt to come to terms with the implications of this changed situation.

Rabinow and Rose (2006: 215) recognise this when they point to the ways in which the politics of health has changed. They ask:

> Who, in 1955, could have imagined depressed people as a global cat-egory, not only as targets but also as active subjects in a new biopolitics of mental health? If we are in an emergent moment of vital politics, celebration or denunciation are insufficient as analytical approaches.

If this is indeed the case, as Gard's paper amply testifies, how can criti-cal intervention happen? What effectivity can it have? Rabinow and Rose (2006: 215) argue that the concept of biopower 'used in a precise fashion, related to empirical investigations and subject to inventive development, would surely have a place as a key part in any analytical toolkit' . . . Is this the case? One of the problems Gard seems to emphasise is that government-based obesity interventions can no longer be countered by critique if that very critique is picked up by groups with very diverse oppositional agendas. In other words, there is no longer a simple politics of opposition, but com-plex oppositional politics with intersecting claims, demands and interests. This would suggest that what is needed to intervene in this field is therefore not only an understanding of power relations and modes of subjectifica-tion as Rabinow and Rose put it, but an engagement with how knowledge circulates globally and is picked up and worked with and over differently in complex intersecting ways. If we take a concept such as Arendt's (1998) web of relations (Studdert 2006) or Mitchell's (1988) relational matrix, how far do these help us to think about the complex relationalities created and constantly shifting which are at work in this and other fields? It would seem from Gard's analysis, that what is at work is a web or matrix of inter-secting vectors, forces or relations. It therefore behoves us to understand how this works in order to develop affective political engagement with such a situation. In this regard, the work of social theorists (e.g. Jervis 1998), which suggests that we cannot know the directions that things will take or the creative outcomes seems particularly important.

With this in mind, let us look at the concept of biopedagogy used in this volume. Of course, as many chapters demonstrate, it captures nicely the pedagogic aspect of biopower, demonstrating its range and force in which everything becomes pedagogized, a work on the self, on the children, on the family and is not simply about school relations. My main issue here is to think about the ways in which we might develop and extend these notions by understanding what happens in relation to what people actually do. This seems to me crucial if we are to understand the complexities raised by Gard's analysis. While Foucault and Foucauldians have worked on texts, apart from work on the discursive organisation of self-management tech-niques, there is little attention to experience or subjectivity as understood in more recent writings (cf Blackman, Cromby, Hook, Papapdopoulos and Walkerdine 2008). So, for example, many of the young women that Geneviève Rail interviewed understood health and fat loss in terms of beauty. In other words, they worked on the self but not in the mode of government targets. So this suggests to me that a relation between the effectivity of biopower and the subject working on the self, or resisting, is too simplistic. Is discourse the only or even best way to understand this? If beauty comes into play, is it simply a discourse of beauty or should we understand how beauty and health work off each other and circulate affectively within the practices in which these young people exist? At the very least we could say that beauty and health work in complex ways to produce subjectivity and that we cannot just read subjectivity off from biopolitical modes of regulation. While the argument in the past has been that subjects are produced through power/knowledge/desire, this suggests a simple relation between regulation and a subject, which is made at least more complex and problematic by the issues of the circulation of knowledge discussed above. These would seem to suggest that even thinking about powers and resistances may be too simplistic. Indeed, Simone Fullagar makes this clear in her analysis of interviews with three families in Queensland. While each family does indeed struggle with weight issues, they do so in different ways and in relation to what Fullagar calls different regimes of meaning. While Fullagar nicely demonstrates for us the affective relations involved, I would like to take this a bit further by pointing to the anxiety about weight loss experienced by the women, their sense of failure, guilt and responsibility, through which their disciplining of themselves and their families has to be accomplished. We also need to note the different circumstances of the families, from concerns about sexuality to fears about lack of safety. Therefore, not only can we not read off the details of the regulative practices and modes of self management from the regulative discourses themselves, but those modes of regulation enter into different communities of practice (Lave and Wenger 1991) and in them different relations of affect. I want particularly to comment on the ways in which responsibilities, fears, guilts, anxieties fall onto the shoulders of the mothers. Moreover, some families used exercise as a form of bonding or togetherness rather than necessarily for health reasons. In that sense, we could say that the affective circulation of the concerns about health and its regulation passes through the figure of the mothers in ways which are consonant with the production of practices of feminine nurturance. Yet, we could not read off what each family did, nor could we automatically read off their desires, concerns or anxieties and the flow and mobilisation of these in practices. While Rabinow and Rose (2006: 215) talk of 'local obstacles and incitements', is this enough in its implication that local things just get in the way or promote specificities while leaving the general analysis intact? What I am exploring rather is the sense that the take-up of regulative discourses and practices around weight and health is complex and indeed cannot be predicted in any simple fashion.

Moreover, the communities of practice and of affect (Walkerdine, 2008), into which these modes of regulation enter, operate in complex ways so that affect circulates relationally through individual bodies, family bodies, community bodies, in ways that we cannot easily predict using a standard governmentality framework. This means that we need other ways of understanding how its effectivities are lived, which suggests, as Doreen Massey (2005) put it, the bringing back of the central importance of politics.

In my own work with ex-steel communities in South Wales, affect could be said to circulate in the affective practices which bind the community together. These are both the arrangements of time and space—hours of working, architecture of terraces of houses, for example, and the ways in which practices build around these to affectively produce a sense of belonging and ontological security (Walkerdine 2008). While these practices might be said to be affected by neoliberal practices of the self, their emergence can be charted by a history of settlement and work in the area, the conditions necessary to withstand harsh working conditions and so forth. In that sense, they move in relation to neoliberal modes of regulation but cannot be predicted by them. The mode of analysis we need, therefore, needs to take these on board just as Fullagar's families had developed their own affective and material practices through which as she put it, their family identities were created.

Annemarie Jutel cites a family who say that without much money to spend on food, a portion of chips is filling. Chips re-appear in Lisette Burrows' children song and in the example of British working class parents putting fish and chips through the playground railings at lunchtime to counter the 'healthy' meals proposed by a recent campaign. How do chips form an assemblage (Deleuze and Guattari 1985) within these different practices? Chips are a predominantly, at least in the British context, white working class food, cheap and filling and also classified as unhealthy. We could therefore analyse how chips function within these various examples, of course though differently but in overlapping ways, which would take us beyond a simple sense that chips function as resistance. Clearly issues of class antagonisms, of comfort, of authority, all appear in these examples. In particular in Murray's chapter (Chapter 6) we see that working class families are understood as not autonomous enough or insufficiently appropriately agentic to work on the self in the correct way. Poor people, she tells us, are thought not to make the right choices and so those have to be made for them. This presents us with the centrality of different modes of regulation for class and poverty, race and ethnicity, fat and thin. The already pathologized subject is not treated in the same way at all as responsive and responsible subject. Thus, the modes of regulation are different. As Helen Lucey and I argued in *Democracy in the Kitchen* (Walkerdine and Lucey 1989), those who cannot reason are at least expected to be reasonable. How then can we think about the regulation of otherness, including the working class, poor, race and ethnicity? In *Democracy in the Kitchen*, we argued that the regulation of mothers was differentiated through their engagement with authority and experience of work and money. Working class mothers in this study (which is admittedly 20 years old now, but nevertheless might give us some pointers) were more likely than their middle class counterparts to separate work and play, to enforce their authority through statements which implied that certain things could or could not be done simply because of their authority and to emphasise the strong relation between adult work and family money. Is it the case then that current approaches in various countries to the issue of obesity assume a liberal subject of autonomy, reason and choice, for whom the poor are always already considered pathological. Does Lisette Burrow's work therefore show us some aspects of the ways in which the poor are objects of something other than agentic biopower? Rather, they have to be made to do certain things, to engage in certain practices 'for their own good'. But, like children singing a song about fish and chips, we cannot control or know the consequences of these interventions.

What is being made and created within these spaces? If we don't simply gloss it as resistance it may be possible to understand these as sites of creation in which something we had not imagined might emerge. While Foucauldian work itself stressed the productivity of modes regulation in the production of subjects, current work deriving from and relating to the rhizomatics of Deleuze and Guattari (2004) stresses creativity and productivity in a different way. That is, creativity evolves (Bergson 1911). The work proposes that something is created which cannot be predicted, unlike Foucault's sense that discourse itself is productive of subject positions which are the only ways that subjects who are the object of biopower can exist. This suggests that within this complex scenario, which Michael Gard laid out so well, we cannot know in advance what will be created form an intervention. We cannot predict totally its effectivity. This makes it both more complex and more hopeful, as those who have suggested that this provides a new space for political action have suggested (Massey 2005).

EMBODIMENT

I want to turn next to Samantha Murray's exploration of the role of medical confession in relation to the fat body. She exemplifies how this creates a set of concerns for fat people about visiting doctors who will always pathologize the weight. This allows us to understand regulative practices as actions upon the body's experience of itself (Bergson, 1911). How is this sensation experienced and how is the pathologized body lived? What can be felt? What is too painful to feel? I suggest we can explore the experience of fat/thin embodiment. Many of the papers do this of course, but I suggest that we need to take this exploration further in future work because in order to think about the complex relationalities into which responses to government policy enter, it is vital to engage with the experience of embodiment. As well as exploring the centrality of unintended consequences of attempts at neoliberal regulation, I want to explore one more issue, raised for me by Emma Rich and John Evan's paper. That is, the different idea of 'voicing' that they put forward. They allow us to think about what can be spoken, but I would like to take that a stage further by thinking about what cannot be and is not spoken. In this way, I want to open up for us to think about the issue of the body's knowledge, what the psychoanalyst Christopher Bollas (1987) calls the 'unthought known'. This is the bodily knowledge that cannot be articulated even if felt and yet the body recognises it; the recognition, for example, of the sensation of disgust, humiliation and what this produces for the body. We can have a 'feeling', from a sensation, a pain, an anxiety, for example, which may be persistent but which cannot be spoken because it cannot be named or known through thought. That is why Bollas calls it the unthought known. If we think about the affective this way, we need to engage with bodies and embodiment in ways which move us beyond constellations of meaning, discourses, practices or creative flows of affect. This approach allows us to engage with embodiment in a different way, but one, I suggest, which is central if we are to be able to take the issue of weight and obesity seriously. These kinds of affects are approached through phenomenology (Merleau Ponty 2002) but also by certain approaches to psychoanalysis. For example, it is quite common for an analyst to experience in her/his own body that which the client feels yet cannot bear to experience (Frosh 2007; Mitrani 2008). In this sense then affect is relational and relationally experienced and dispersed. It is only by patient work and an embodied sense of safety that the embodied knowledge may be thought. In other words then, there is an aspect of embodiment which cannot be approached through discursive and textual analyses but which may have a central place in understanding fat and thin bodies and the experiences of regulation. In some research that I have been undertaking in South Wales, some young unemployed men refused to take available work, mostly working in supermarkets, because they considered it embarrassing and feminine. What emerged from the research is that these feelings were moving in a dynamic way between members of the community and the young men. By this I mean that many family members and workmates of both sexes made them feel feminised if they took such work. Female workmates called a young man 'Mrs Mop' when he worked with them as a cleaner; a father refused to talk to his son when he had to dress up in a uniform while working for Domino's Pizza.

Interview data and an understanding of the community history led to the conclusion that the sense of shame and humiliation experienced by the young men was projected onto them because they appeared to embody the shameful end to a mode of masculine labour in which there had been generations of pride. The distress that community members felt about its loss and their inability to pass on something good to their children, was unconsciously projected onto these young men who experienced the feelings that the rest of the community could not bear to feel. I understand that this mode of explanation does use notions of an unconscious, but what I am more wanting to point to are the complex relationalities through which affect circulates, so that when we are dealing with the experience of fat or thin bodies this may be manifest in ways which require complex modes of explanation which understand the dynamics of affective relations. The problem was, therefore not the young men but the pain, shame and humiliation circulating within the community. In order to understand this, it was necessary to infer it from what was not said and then to take it back as a working hypothesis to the community members themselves.

In the same vein, therefore, I am suggesting there is an unspoken other to the subject of biopower. The subject of choice, freedom, hides, elides and defends against its other, that which neoliberalism itself cannot bear to utter, cannot bear to face. Just as Rail's subjects chose beauty over health, so each of the aspects of the neoliberal subject has that which is elided, split off, disavowed. Where does it go? What is the Other of neoliberalism that has to be so strongly regulated for fear that it may break out? We have seen its emergence in the families who must be reasonable because they are deemed unable to reason. In this sense, a set of affective relations circulates around or beneath the regulative practices. Here we can see bodies out of control, whose costs in terms of illness cannot be borne by state regulated health services. We see bodies who refuse to regulate themselves. This directs us to the anxieties which act as the vital drivers of these initiatives, which need themselves to be understood and addressed rather than simply understanding a force as a will to power and truth. This opens up a concern with the anxieties of government which cannot be spoken as well as the desires for profit unarticulated in each new commercial initiative, each new slimming product. So, my proposal is that these anxieties circulate through the lifeworld. They are experienced both in the practices and policies and in the communities, families and individual bodies. The more the unthought known of all these areas can be brought to light the more it can be addressed. In this sense I am attempting to introduce a note of complexity. Just because something is not included as the subject of biopower does not mean that it is not there! Rather it suggests a massive anxiety about its possible appearance. But it is being denied. I felt that this emerged in different ways in every single paper.

'When my body starts to disappear. People start to see me', says one of the girls in Rich and Evan's research. In other words, only the slim female body can be 'seen'—the aim is not to be noticed as a fat girl but as an attractive slim girl. The truism that inside every fat body is a thin one trying to get out, speaks of affective conflict, an embodied struggle to be seen, to be heard, to belong, to be liked, to be accepted and held, to be safe. These are complex affective issues which are barely being addressed by the subject who is object of these regimes. This subject knows, controls, acts, is responsible for themselves. What an impoverished and simplistic subject this is. What about the ill or pathologised bodies for whom illness or pathology are the only ways of 'saying' something which cannot be articulated or perhaps thought any other way? What and how does the body speak? What is the fat or thin body speaking? How do we read such bodies—through love, hate, anxiety, wanting, needing, shame, delight? What is distressed and how can distress be articulated? The biopedagogic technologies produce a vision of a Robinson Crusoe subject adrift from the relationalities through which it was formed and only responsible for itself. Every study cited in this volume showed this to be a completely inadequate way of understanding the issues.

If I may manage a small personal example: I go to the local gym to train, but I am often aware that alongside me so to speak in training is a fat girl who was frightened of her body, who was full of self hatred and who felt that she was unlovable. This girl longs to feed and be fed but the slim toned body must make sure no trace of her can be seen, even if an emotional battle is played out over the surface of the body, through the apparatus of the gym, in the choice of meals to be made. That other is always there in the background. What then if we were to let in the other of biopower, the other of the regulated body. What bodies would emerge from the shadows? Are those bodies so terrifyingly grotesque that we have to banish them from our sights forever?

Yet just like the fat girl of my imagination and my childhood history, those others are already there stalking the practices as a ghost walks at midnight. The relations through which those bodies are formed are also present as so much work in this book testifies. In that sense then it is the relationalities we need to explore. The anthropologist Thomas Csordas (1994) tells us that before the conquest of the Americas, for the indigenous worldview, there was no singular body and no way to articulate it. What I take him to mean is that bodies were connected in complex ways and that there was no focus on the regulation of a singular body who could be observed, known. This is what came with the colonial gaze. The postmodern neoliberal gaze focuses on singular subjects, but if we put those subjects back into the relationalities that form them, we see a different picture (Walkerdine 2007). If we refuse to separate figure and ground, we see relations themselves and it is those we can analyse to find what Deleuze and Guattari (1985) named an assemblage or Hannah Arendt a 'who' (Studdert, 2006). This is not the same as an embodied person, but a constellation of relations that are moving and temporary.

This collection of papers makes an excellent introduction to critical work on biopolitical issues around weight and obesity. This is a crucial political topic that deserves to be further developed. The complex politics of today and the paths discussed by the papers in this volume attest to the urgent need to find new modes of analysis and new practices of intervention which are adequate to the current conjuncture. This is daunting but exciting work.

REFERENCES

Arendt, H. (1998) *The Human Condition*, Chicago: University of Chicago Press.

Bergson, H. (1911) *Creative Evolution*, London: Macmillan.

Blackman, L., Cromby, J., Hook, D.W., Papapdopoulos, D. and Walkerdine, V. (2008) 'Editorial: Creating Subjectivities', *Subjectivity*, 22: 1–27

Bollas, C. (1987) *The Shadow of the Object: Psychoanalysis of the Unthought Unknown*, London: Free Association Books.

Csordas, T. (1994) *Embodiment and Experience*, Cambridge: Cambridge University Press.

Deleuze, G. and Guattari, G. (1985) *Anti-Oedipus*, London: Athlone.

Deleuze, G. and Guattari, F. (2004) *A Thousand Plateaus*, London: Continuum

Frosh, S. (2007) 'Affect and encounter', *Critical Psychology*, 21: 76–93.

Gard, M. and Wright, J. (2005) *The Obesity Epidemic: Science, Morality and Ideology*, London: Routledge.

Jervis, R. (1998) *System Effects: Complexity in Political and Social Life*, Princeton: Princeton University Press.

Lave, J. and Wenger, E. (1991) *Situated Learning: Legitimate Peripheral Participation*, Cambridge: Cambridge University Press.

Massey, D. (2005) *For Space*, London: Sage.

Merleau Ponty, M. (2002) *Phenomenology of Perception*, London: Routledge.

Mitchell, S. (1988) *Relational Concepts in Psychoanalysis*, Cambridge Mass: Harvard University Press.

Mitrani, J. (2008) *A Framework for the Imaginary*, London: Karnac.

Rabinow, P. and Rose, N. (2006) 'Biopower today', *BioSocieties*, 1: 195–217.

Studdert, D.H. (2006) *Conceptualising Community: Beyond the State and the Individual*, Basingstoke: Palgrave.

Urry, J. (2003) *Global Complexity*, Oxford: Polity.

Walkerdine, V. (2007) *Children, Gender, Videogames: Towards a Relational Approach to Multimedia*, Basingstoke: PalgraveMacmillan.

Walkerdine, V. (2008) 'Communities of Affect', paper presented at the *Subjectivity International Conference*, Cardiff University, June 2008.

Walkerdine, V. and Lucey, H. (1989) *Democracy in the Kitchen*, London: Virago.

Contributors

Laura Azzarito is a lecturer and researcher in the School of Sport and Exercise Sciences at Loughborough University. Her current research includes an ethnographic project which explores young people's narratives of their physicality in non-traditional physical education curriculum, and an historical project which aims to understand the links among American schooling, physical education curriculum, fatness, and health discourses between the 1950s and the 1970s.

Natalie Beausoleil is Associate Professor of Social Science and Health, Faculty of Medicine, University of New Foundland. She has published extensively on women's health (and specifically eating disorders and body image, and is currently working on research focusing on the discursive constructions of the body, health, and fitness among youth in Canada.

Lisette Burrows is a Associate Professor in physical education at the School of Physical Education, University of Otago. Her research is informed by poststructuralist social theory and critical psychology and is focused on the deconstruction of curriculum initiatives, empirical understandings of young people's engagement with physical culture and health and a critical interrogation of developmental discourses in the social construction of formal and informal health and physical education.

John Evans is Professor of Sociology of Education and Physical Education in the School of Sport and Exercise Sciences. His research interests centre on issues relating to the politics of the curriculum, equity and identity, in relation to physical education. His current research focuses on the relationships between education and eating disorders. Most recently, with Emma Rich Brian Davies and Rachel Allwood, he has co-authored the Routledge publication, *Obesity, Education and Eating Disorders: fat fabrications.*

Simone Fullagar is a senior lecturer and interdisciplinary sociologist in the Department of Tourism, Leisure, Hotel and Sport Management at Griffith University, Queensland, Australia. Drawing upon post-structuralist, feminist and governmental perspectives she has published widely within international journals within the sociology of health and leisure. Her most recent project examines how different families and active living policy makers take up or refuse current discourses about healthy life-styles in the context of the 'obesity epidemic'.

Michael Gard is an Associate Professor at Charles Sturt University who has an established international reputation as a researcher, writer and commentator in the area of social research, policy and school practice on the 'obesity epidemic'. He has written widely for scholarly and popular audiences about obesity and is a regular electronic media commentator on the obesity panic. Most recently, his work has focused on the political and ideological dimensions of anti-obesity public policy. He is lead author of *The Obesity Epidemic: Science, Morality and Ideology* published by Routledge.

Christine Halse is Professor of Education and Director of the Centre for Educational Research at the University of Western Sydney. She is a sociologist of education who teaches and researches in the areas of educational policy, qualitative research, and educational evaluation. She is internationally know for her use of life history methods, and has recently completed a large-scale, multi-disciplinary study of the experiences of teenage girls and parents living with anorexia nervosa. She is lead author of *Inside Anorexia: The Experiences of Girls and Their Families* (JKP 2008).

Valerie Harwood is a senior lecturer in the Faculty of Education at the University of Wollongong. Her research focus is on youth and psycho-pathologisation. She has recently published a book, *Diagnosing 'Disorderly' Children* (2006, Routledge), which examines the associations made between young people, marginalisation and psychopathology. Her current research focuses on the ADHD phenomenon and disadvantage.

Annemarie Jutel is an Associate Professor of nursing and midwifery at Otago Polytechnic in Dunedin, New Zealand. She has published extensively on critical topics surrounding the size of the body. Her work has focused on the historical values that lead society to attach labels to body size, the place of medicine in reinforcing those values by diagnostic categories, and the gendered nature of preoccupation with body size and appearance. She has published in journals such as *Perspectives in Biology and Medicine, Healthy Weight Networks, Social Science and Medicine* and *Social Semiotics*.

Deana Leahy is a lecturer at Southern Cross University, Australia. Her research interests include historical and sociocultural analyses of policy/curriculum and pedagogy within health education, education and health promotion more broadly. Her work is largely informed by Foucauldian inspired writings around governmentality.

Samantha Murray is a Postdoctoral Research Fellow in the Somatechnics Research Centre/Department of Critical and Cultural Studies at Macquarie University, Sydney, Australia. She is the author of *The 'Fat' Female Body* (Palgrave Macmillan, 2008), co-editor with Nikki Sullivan of *Somatechnics: Queering the Technologisation of Bodies* (forthcoming in 2009, Ashgate), and has published numerous articles on the discursive constructions of embodiment, normalcy and pathology.

Geneviève Rail is Professor in the Faculty of Health Sciences at the University of Ottawa and co-Chair of the Center for Critical Research in Health. Her research interests focus on the sociocultural study of physical activity, the body and health. She is well known as a feminist critic of body-related institutions (e.g. sport, media, health systems and industries) and favors queer, poststructuralist and postcolonial approaches. She is currently involved in a series of funded research projects focusing on young Canadian women's discursive constructions of health and obesity.

Emma Rich is a senior lecturer in Gender Identity Health and Physical Education in the School of Sport and Exercise Sciences, Loughborough University. She is currently involved in a number of projects exploring the relationships between education and ill health, with a particular focus on eating disorders. Conceptually much of her work is informed by sociological, educational and feminist theory drawing upon qualitative methodologies. She is co-author of the books, *The Medicalisation of Cyberspace*, with Andy Miah and *Obesity, Education and Eating Disorders* with John Evans, Brian Davies and Rachel Allwood.

Valerie Walkerdine is a research Professor at the University of Cardiff, Wales. She has published extensively in the areas of critical psychology, young people and popular culture and psychosocial explorations of gender and class. Her most recent books include (with Blackman) *Mass Hysteria: Critical Psychology and Media Studies, Children, gender, video games: towards a relational approach to multimedia,* and Walkerdine (with Lucey and Melody) *Growing Up Girl: Gender & Class in the 21st Century.*

Jan Wright is research Professor of Education in the Faculty of Education at the University of Wollongong. Her research draws on feminist and poststructuralist theory to critically engage issues associated with the relationship between embodiment, culture and health. Her most recent work has focused on social constructions of youth, particularly in the context of public health imperatives and schooling. She is co-editor of *Body Knowledge and Control and Critical Inquiry* and *Problem Solving in Physical Education* (Routledge 2004) and co-author with Michael Gard of *The Obesity Epidemic: Science, Ideology and Morality* (Routledge 2005).

Index

NB: 'n' after a page number refers to a note.